COMMUNITY STEWARDSHIP

Applying the Five Principles of

CONTEMPORARY GOVERNANCE

Scott W. Goodspeed

14107

AHA
Press

An American Hospital Association Company
Chicago

Cover Design by Jeanne Calabrese

Library of Congress Cataloging-in-Publication Data

Goodspeed, Scott W.
    Community stewardship : applying the five principles of
contemporary governance / Scott W. Goodspeed.
        p.   cm.
    Includes bibliographical references and index.
    1. Hospitals—Administration.   2. Hospital trustees.   3. Hospital
and community.   I. Title.
RA971.G59   1997
362.1'1'068—dc21   97-28475
                                                                   CIP

ISBN: 1-55648-210-8   Item Number: 196228

COMMUNITY STEWARDSHIP

Applying the Five Principles of
Contemporary Governance

Contents

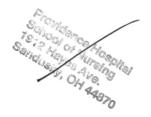

CHAPTER 4

The Five Core Competencies of Highly Effective Boards

Community Stewardship   •   Visionary Leadership   •
Systems Thinking   •   High-Leverage Actions   •
Basic Business Skills   •   Conclusion

About the Author

Scott W. Goodspeed, F.A.C.H.E., is president and CEO of Goodspeed, a national management consulting firm in Bedford, New Hampshire, aspiring to create healthy futures for individuals, organizations, communities, and nations. The firm specializes in strategic planning, community stewardship, executive coaching, and 21st-century governance. Before founding Goodspeed, he was the president and CEO of a 300-bed community hospital, vice president and COO of a $300 million health care system, and president and CEO of an academic medical center.

Mr. Goodspeed holds a bachelor's degree in administration of health care services from Ithaca College, Ithaca, New York, and a masters of hospital administration from the University of Minnesota, Minneapolis.

Mr. Goodspeed has served on over 20 nonprofit boards and has authored articles on strategic planning, governance, and quality improvement. He has delivered numerous presentations to various professional associations and health care systems on strategic planning, community stewardship, and 21st-century governance.

He is the recipient of a number of professional awards and honors including The Healthcare Forum and Korn/Ferry International 1992 Emerging Leaders in Healthcare Award, The Healthcare Forum's 1993 Creating Healthier Communities Fellowship, the 1994 *Modern Healthcare*/Governance Institute Governance Fellowship Award, and the 1996 American Leadership Forum Fellowship. He is a recipient of the 1997–1998 Who's Who in Medicine and Healthcare, Marquis Who's Who, New Providence, New Jersey.

Think not forever of yourselves, O Chiefs,
nor of your own generation.

Think of continuing generations of our families,
think of your grandchildren
and of those yet unborn,
Whose faces are coming from
beneath the ground.

—*The Peacemaker,*
  founder of the Iroquois Confederacy,
  circa *1000* A.D.

Preface

A silent revolution is going on across the country. In every state, healthy community initiatives are gaining momentum. Every health care organization has the opportunity to improve its governance and to facilitate community initiatives that contribute significantly to community health status. *Community Stewardship* presents a more effective governance system and a new set of core competencies geared toward the creation of healthy communities.

RESPONDING TO THE ENVIRONMENT

A profound set of changes is occurring around us, and the pace of change has far exceeded governance practices. Board responsibility can take many forms, depending on the organization and the environment. Sometimes, it means governance taking the initiative when government has gotten caught up in legislative gridlock. Along the same lines, responsibility can mean being alert to opportunities put forth by corporations or organizations that share a board's interest in community health. One such opportunity came in 1994 when the American Hospital Association, the Catholic Health Association of the United States, VHA Inc., and The Hospital Research and Educational Trust jointly announced a $6 million grant from the W. K. Kellogg Foundation to realize the vision of Community Care Networks[SM] (CCNs) across the country. The vision pushes for simultanous achievement of four goals:

- community health focus
- community accountability
- seamless continuum of care
- management within fixed resources[1]

As the project unfolded, Kellogg was joined by the Duke Endowment, the U.S. Public Health Service, the Robert Wood Johnson Foundation, and others. Almost 300 organizations, hospitals, and health networks applied for the grant money, and from this number 25 sites were selected as awardees, including the Southcentral Health Network of Idaho's Healthy Communities 2000 project described in chapter 4 of this book.

Governance responsibility demands that boards not only understand the changes that may have a positive or negative influence on the organization but that they anticipate and respond to external influences in a proactive manner. Many of these external influences also have an impact on communities. How health care organizations respond has an effect on the communities they serve. The best way to respond is to make sure that a system of governance is in place that recognizes that our organizations are really part of something larger and that the progress we make in health care will be part of progress we make on many fronts. To renew our governance practices, boards need to lay the foundations of 21st-century governance and to lead systemic change in their communities.

GOVERNANCE PRINCIPLES FOR THE NEW CENTURY

A set of governance principles developed over the last century has laid the groundwork for how we govern our health care organizations. These principles have enabled boards to preserve the order already in place. It is time to set aside these principles and adopt a new set of governance principles that will enable a new order to emerge. This book is about a way of governing health care organizations that will profoundly change America's health care landscape. The new governance principles focus on collaboration and acknowledge the importance of creating and building healthy communities. Collaboration has replaced competition as the byword of health care. Among the applicants to the CCN demonstration project described above, those that became awardees indicated that, on average, just over one-half of their services are provided or produced collaboratively.

Board members from across the country are beginning to realize that systemic change is emerging. One board chair from California said to me, "Think *community*, rather than *my hospital*." A board chair from Wisconsin suggested, "Understand the role of governance. The goal should be to help integrate for a cost-effective, healthy community, not to protect your institution. If necessary, be a leader and close your hospital down rather than try to ineffectively compete." A board chair in New Jersey advised, "Assess community needs, collaborate with all health organizations, and stop duplication of services."

TARGET READERSHIP

This book is principally for trustees of hospitals and health care systems who are interested in improving the health of their communities and in effective governance. CEOs, physician executives, planners, business and industry leaders, and community-based organizations that have a vision of creating a healthy community will also find the book useful. *Community Stewardship* makes the case for creating healthy communities, identifies the governance leadership gap, proposes a more effective way of governing, and provides experience-based guidance through the use of case examples and stories spread throughout the book.

THE EFFECTIVE GOVERNANCE SYSTEM

There are three building blocks in the effective governance system. Each building block alone is not enough to create and sustain healthy communities long term. Altogether, they form a durable and sturdy model. Figure 1 shows the model of the effective governance system that is developed in detail over the course of this book.

The Five Principles of Contemporary Governance

The five principles of contemporary governance are at the base of the pyramid because they provide the anchor for creating and building healthy communities. All of the governance decisions are fundamentally rooted in these five principles. Boards need to challenge many of their old assumptions about their belief structure and gain clarity around the five principles of contemporary governance. These principles become

FIGURE 1. The Effective Governance System

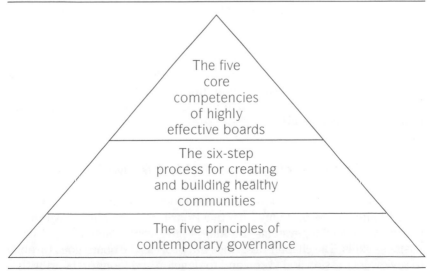

The five
core
competencies
of highly
effective boards

The six-step
process for creating
and building healthy
communities

The five principles of
contemporary governance

part of a new belief system and provide overall guidance for all operational, strategic, and community health care decisions. These principles initially are acted upon consciously, and over time they become a routine part of what the organization stands for and strives for.

On the basis of these five principles, chapter 1, "Moving from Trusteeship to Governance Team Stewardship," makes some claims about governance in the 21st century: Trusteeship will diminish in importance and governance team stewardship will arise in its place. Twenty-first-century governance will embody a broader and more active spirit. Governance teams will focus on both the health of their organization and the health of the populations they serve. They will operate under a new definition of health and a new definition of governance.

Chapter 2, "Taking the Path to the Healthy Community," defines a healthy community and discusses the emerging model of collaboration. Collaboration and community learning will transcend organizational needs in the 21st century. The chapter offers three different frameworks for creating healthy communities, and once these frameworks are understood, governance teams are ready to start creating healthy communities.

The Six-Step Process for Creating and Building Healthy Communities

The six-step process for creating and building healthy communities is the second building block of the pyramidal model for 21st-century governance. The process gives boards a methodology to gain commitment and initiate action toward creating healthy communities. It helps to organize our thinking about how boards learn and how to work with others to create healthier communities. Chapter 3, "The Six-Step Process for Creating and Building Healthy Communities," describes the model in detail.

There is a strong correlation between an organization's ability to create and build healthy communities and the effectiveness of its governance. Most effective boards have adopted a system of governance that helps sustain the healthy community vision. The third building block for 21st-century governance contains the five core competencies of highly effective boards.

The Five Core Competencies of Highly Effective Boards

Chapter 4 defines and explores the third block of the pyramid, "The Five Core Competencies of Highly Effective Boards": community stewardship, visionary leadership, systems thinking, high-leverage actions, and basic business skills. The chapter describes the process the board goes through to review its mission and vision and to develop and monitor its priorities.

In time, boards will redefine their core business and focus on both keeping people well and their community's quality-of-life issues. Mastery of the core competencies has specific and identifiable consequences in the practice of health care delivery, and case studies and board testimony illuminate some those consequences.

Scattered throughout the book are brief quotations, written by actual board members from across the country. These quotes should help the reader to reflect on the leadership challenges that we all face as we attempt to guide our organizations into the 21st century.

Community Stewardship closes with an epilogue that demonstrates how the effective governance system converges with Peter Senge's concept of the learning organization and that provides a governance profile that board members can use as a self-test. The book also contains two appendixes. The first presents the findings of a research report I made titled "21st Century Governance: Competencies of Highly Successful Boards." The report was made possible by the 1994 Governance Fellowship Award given to me by The Governance Institute in La Jolla, California, and *Modern Healthcare* magazine. The second appendix contains the healthy community contract, which was designed to recognize the board's commitment to community stewardship. The bibliography of this book contains one section for each of the five core competencies of highly successful boards.

COMMUNITY STEWARDSHIP: THE BIG PICTURE

In the world economy, cities and communities will emerge as important players. We must understand the relationship between our organizations and the social context that surrounds them. In the 21st century, we will see regional collaboration, the rebirth of community consciousness, governance team stewardship, and more effective governance. The problems facing the health care system are urgent. Those health care organizations that proceed down the paths leading to healthy communities and effective governance will develop sustainable practices and lead systemic change in health care.

Reference

1. Richard Bogue and Claude H. Hall Jr., *Health Network Innovations: How 20 Communities Are Improving Their Systems through Collaboration* (Chicago: American Hospital Publishing, 1997), p. xxix.

Acknowledgments

T his book took more than two years from conception to completion. I am indebted to the many organizations and board members
for their encouragement, advice, and thoughts. This book could
not have been created without their help.

I especially wish to acknowledge the following:

- Richard Hill, senior editor, American Hospital Publishing, Inc., for providing guidance and support. This book reflects his editorial wisdom and considerable talent.
- Pat Fiene, development editor, American Hospital Publishing, Inc., for her considerable support and talent, which made the book more reader-friendly.
- Charlie Ewell, president and CEO of The Governance Institute, and *Modern Healthcare*, for awarding me the Governance Fellowship Award, which funded the research on 21st-century governance.
- VHA Inc., The Catholic Health Association of the United States, and Anthony R. Kovner, Ph.D., from New York University's Robert F. Wagner Graduate School of Public Service, for having the wisdom to develop their frameworks for community benefit and the kindness to share them with others.
- Richard J. Davidson, president, American Hospital Association, and the AHA board, for having the vision and insight to support "a society of healthy communities, where all individuals reach their highest potential for health."
- Kathryn E. Johnson, president and CEO of The Healthcare Forum, and The Healthcare Forum Board, who introduced me to the healthy community vision.
- Gregory Javornisky, Ph.D., and Danielle Marie Chenelle, who provided considerable research advice and talent interpreting the results of the governance health care survey.
- Pam Tomazic, who typed and retyped this manuscript from start to finish. Her commitment to this project was invaluable.

- Fawn Peterson and Becky Phillips, my administrative assistants, for keeping everything else going while this book was being written.
- My wife, Mary-Ellen, and our two children, Katie and Brendan, to whom this book is dedicated. They deserve special thanks for tolerating the endless hours I spent writing this book.

1

Moving from Trusteeship to Governance Team Stewardship

The journey of a thousand miles begins with one step.

—*Lao Tzu*

There must be a better way to govern our health care organizations in the 21st century. During my discussions with board chairs across the country, one overriding concern became clear: Trustees need a more meaningful and compelling connection to their health care organization and community. John Carver writes, in his important book, *Boards That Make a Difference:*

> Board members arrive at the table with dreams. They have vision and values. Yet, by and large, board members do not spend their time exploring, debating, and defining those dreams. Instead, they expend their energy on a host of demonstrably less important, even trivial, items. Instead of impassioned discussion about the change to be produced in their world, board members are ordinarily found passively listening to staff reports. Most of what the majority of boards do either does not need to be done or is a waste of time when done by the board.[1]

A few examples illustrate the need for boards to connect with their communities:

- In a medium-size community, the merger and consolidation of two community hospitals begins to disintegrate. The board chair says, "This was our hope, our dream, and our vision. We focused on our traditional board agenda and functions and we somehow lost our connection to the community."
- The board of a health care organization located in a large urban community discovers that the community's infant mortality rate is higher

than that of some third world countries. The board chair says, "Why did we have to read about this in a national newspaper? How can this be? We have the most resources, skills, and capabilities in the world, yet our neighbors receive the worst care in the world."

- In a small, rural community, a group of citizens forms an association to seek better ways of gaining access to primary care. The past board chair of the local community hospital, frustrated because the local hospital would not get involved, leads the association, which opens a clinic that competes with the community hospital.

As a result of these experiences, the boards of the organizations in these examples began to question their beliefs and values. More important, they began to explore their roles, to debate the extent to which their organizations were meeting the needs of the community, and to have impassioned discussions about their real purpose—to be stewards of community health. Trustees need and want this more meaningful connection with their communities. One board chair said to me, "We are missing something so fundamental—our commitment to create healthy communities."

This chapter presents both economic and altruistic reasons for making the transition from traditional trusteeship to governance team stewardship. It identifies five principles that will guide governance in the 21st century and describes a variety of successful initiatives based on these principles. The chapter closes with an examination of how a compelling vision can inspire organizations to change.

THE NEED FOR GOVERNANCE TEAM STEWARDSHIP

"We must empower the organization and the community to act collectively to improve the health status of our population."

As we move into the 21st century, both economics and altruism compel us to improve the health of our communities through community stewardship. Almost half of the leading causes of death in the United States are preventable. The development of protocols to manage the course of disease before the disease becomes acute will result in fewer inpatient days and fewer visits to the physician's office. The time spent on the front end preventing death and managing disease means fewer resources consumed on the back end. The managed care environment emphasizes and rewards fiscal responsibility, and the disease prevention and management programs that come about through community stewardship make sound fiscal sense.

Equally important, stewardship of community health will improve the quality of life of those served by providers. The ideal is to go beyond seeing health as the absence of disease and seek to *create* health. This new perspective requires active engagement with communities; exploration of the social and economic conditions that lead to health; and collaboration with the school system, police department, and other community institutions to understand the root issues related to health. If health is more than just the absence of disease, then it includes all the following:

- the promotion of health and disease prevention
- the development of adequate housing
- the reduction of crime
- the promotion of safety
- the creation of employment opportunities
- the eradication of illegal drug activity

In short, as much needs to be done outside the four walls of organizations as inside them.

In a recent book, Peter Block states, "Stewardship begins with the willingness to be accountable for some larger body than ourselves—an organization, a community. Stewardship springs from a set of beliefs about reforming organizations that affirms our choice for service over pursuit of self-interest."[2] Health care governance teams in the 21st century will affirm their choice for service and create healthy populations.

When boards affirm their choice for service, they commit to a course of action whereby their principal concern is for the health of the community they serve. This commitment impels them and their health organizations to act differently. Organizations that have made the transition have begun to

- collaborate with others to achieve a higher quality of life for the community
- adopt information systems that track patterns of disease and promote better management of the incidence of disease in the community
- pursue primary interventions aimed at promoting health and avoiding illness
- revise their vision and mission statements so that stewardship becomes the priority, followed by profit
- revise the board agenda and restructure board activities and functions
- establish a committee dedicated to community health

- adapt their continuous quality improvement processes and indicators to include the work they do in the community

FIVE PRINCIPLES OF 21ST-CENTURY GOVERNANCE

"The old days of 'country-club' trusteeship are over. Boards must use aggressive business strategies to lead their health care institutions along the path to survival."

Trustees hold a unique position in their health care organization. Entrusted with the welfare of their organization and its community, trustees are in the best position to challenge old assumptions and move their organization into a new era of stewardship. As we move into the 21st century, boards need not preserve and protect what currently exists. The United States can no longer afford to spend a large percentage of its gross national product on health care. As the payment system shifts from fee for service to capitation, health care organizations must shift their focus from delivery of sick care to delivery of health care.

Table 1-1 contrasts the major principles by which health care organizations have been governed during this century with principles that will govern organizations in the 21st century. As the table shows, governance during this century has generally been focused inward. Organizations have striven to preserve and protect the current order, have viewed health care as complication management, and have sought to

TABLE 1-1. Governance Principles: 20th Century versus 21st Century

20th century	21st century
Preserve and protect the current order	Create the conditions for a new order to emerge
Define health care as complication management	Redefine health care in terms of disease management and community health
Be mission driven	Become vision and mission driven
Promote self-interest	Promote stewardship
Enable the organization	Empower the organization and the community

fulfill their missions by promoting their own interests. In contrast, 21st-century health care organizations will be focused outward. Driven by a compelling vision and mission, organizations will focus on disease management and the creation of a healthy community and will collaborate with other leaders to empower their communities to create health.

Governance in the 21st century will center on five themes: change, economics, collaboration, possibility, and healthy communities. The governance principles that will create the foundation for 21st-century governance embody these themes.

Principle 1: Create the Conditions for a New Order to Emerge

The first governance principle suggests that boards are already empowered to create the right conditions or environment for a new order; they need only to challenge existing assumptions, to think outside the box, and to mobilize the energy within their boardrooms and organizations. Fulfillment of this first principle means that the board examines what exists and asks *why?* and dreams of a better way and asks *why not?* It reaches out to others in new and different ways. The case examples that follow illustrate how out-of-the-box thinking led to a new order for several health care organizations and their communities.

The Manchester Agenda In Manchester, New Hampshire, in 1993, the Elliot Hospital and the Catholic Medical Center, along with 30 of New Hampshire's business and civic leaders, participated in a community initiative called the Manchester Agenda. With input from all contingents, this group developed a compelling, shared vision of greater Manchester as a collaborative community. The group adopted a set of core community values and commitments, and health care was a part of the agenda: "We work for the health of all of our people through a comprehensive health-care delivery system with a strong emphasis on collaboration and cooperation between healthcare providers and the community, with the ultimate goal of creating a healthy community."[3] This statement of commitment assisted in creating conditions that transformed health care in Manchester. The hospitals jointly participated in the Hospital Community Benefits Standards Program (a national demonstration initiative that assisted health care organizations to develop a systematic community benefit program), built a community health center, and eventually consolidated their organizations' holding companies to create Optima Health, Inc. At the same time, other community leaders focused on revitalizing the local economy, improving education, promoting diversity, and encouraging public-private collaboration. A new organization was established to manage and implement many of the items that came out of the Manchester Agenda. As a result of the initiative, fundamental assumptions that had gone unchallenged were reversed, and the new order that emerged led to better coordination and consolidation of community resources. (See chapter four for more information about the Manchester Agenda.)

The Southside Institutions Neighborhood Alliance In April 1996, the Southside Institutions Neighborhood Alliance (SINA), composed of five organizations located on the south side of Hartford, Connecticut, announced the launch of a comprehensive neighborhood revitalization initiative for Hartford. With the participation of the member institutions—Hartford Hospital, The Institute of Living, Trinity College, the Connecticut Children's Medical Center, and Connecticut Public Television and Radio—the $175 million initiative will create an infrastructure for local families and link neighborhood institutions in an unprecedented collaboration. The initiative includes a kindergarten-through-12th-grade educational component and a science component focusing on health and technology. Three new schools, a new health and technology center, an early childhood and family resource center, and a boys and girls club are to be established in the target area. SINA also entails a comprehensive program for expanding home ownership, creating businesses and jobs, improving education and job skills, and enhancing access to social services to revitalize its needy neighborhoods. Finally, SINA created a new governance structure with a SINA board and executive committee whose sole purpose is to create a healthier community.

In this sterling example of collaboration, a college, a public television station, and three health care organizations redefined their core business, restructured their board's activities, and formed a new organization with its own governance structure and governance team stewardship. In short, out of ordinary discussion came an extraordinary idea, and SINA created the conditions for a better quality of life in Hartford.

Principle 2: Redefine Health Care in Terms of Disease Management and Community Health

The second governance principle challenges boards to rethink their organizations' core business. Health care in the 21st century must be redefined to include disease management, population-based management of care, and the creation of healthy communities.

The disease management concept is based on an examination of the interrelated elements of a disease and the impact of one stage of a disease on later stages. Disease management has shown that in many cases, preventive or corrective action can halt or postpone the progress of a disease. Population-based management of care focuses on covered lives—the number of people in a geographic area enrolled in a health care plan for which the health care organization is responsible. Some boards have redefined their core business to focus on keeping people well and enhancing their quality of life. These boards have also broadened their geographic reach so that their focus is more regional and less local. The two organizations described below have challenged their fundamental core business assumptions.

The Memorial Hospital and Health System In South Bend, Indiana, the Memorial Hospital and Health System committed to making "healthier communities . . . an integral part of the Memorial Hospital Health System mission. In practice, creating healthier communities takes the shape of an array of community health enhancement initiatives to address health issues before they become health problems." Memorial Hospital and Health System community health enhancement initiatives include the following:

- *Urban Care:* A project for collaborative community health care delivery in disadvantaged areas and for a target population with common needs.
- *HealthStart Well Child Clinic:* A preventive medical and dental clinic for children whose parents' income is at or near poverty level.
- *African American Women in Touch (WIT):* A group whose goal is to get the message across that many African American women are needless victims of breast cancer and that many deaths could be avoided by means of cancer prevention and early detection.[4]

As these initiatives show, the Memorial Hospital and Health System redefined and refocused its core business so that healthier communities became an integral part of the system's mission and vision. In addition, the initiatives illustrate the commitment to collaborate with others in the community, to coordinate resources, and to reach out to improve community health.

Northwest Community Healthcare Northwest Community Healthcare (NWCH) in Arlington Heights, Illinois, is a recognized leader in a number of community-based health and wellness initiatives. Its initiatives began with a mission statement, a primary objective, and a board committed to creating a healthy community. NWCH's mission is as follows:

We exist to provide quality, compassionate healthcare services to the people of the northwest community. We are more than a hospital charged with fixing health problems. We are responsible for improving the health of our community from year to year. Every community has a set of social services designed to meet its needs. These generally include police, fire, education, and, in some cases, healthcare. We have been charged via our Mission as the stewards of healthcare for the people in the northwest suburban area.[5]

NWCH provides another compelling example of a health care organization and governance team redefining a key component of core business and doing what is in the best interest of the community.

Principle 3: Become Vision and Mission Driven

The third governance principle suggests that organizations need to shift from being mission driven to being both vision and mission driven. An organization's mission statement defines the organization's purpose and creates the central province within the board's domain. It should reflect reality, focus on ends rather than means, and be understandable. A well-wrought mission statement is important, because it provides guidance for organizational members and influences their behaviors. But a mission statement alone is not enough. The mission must be driven by a compelling vision of where the organization aspires to be. A compelling vision puts a stake in the ground some time in the future, and it is both manageable and measurable. The vision determines how the organization governs in the future and how it views all future relationships. The organizations described in the following case examples are guided by inspiring visions.

Health Partners of Southern Arizona In Tucson, Arizona, the health care system Health Partners of Southern Arizona held a Healthier Tucson Community Forum dedicated to improving the health status of the community. Broad community participation provided a new source of input into its vision. The Community Forum is a collaborative effort. It was initiated and sponsored locally by a number of organizations, including Tucson Medical Center, Tucson newspapers, and United Way; and nationally by The Healthcare Forum with support from the National Civic League. Healthier Tucson brought together a diverse group of community leaders (80 to 100 who represent various segments and interests within the community) to address and respond to Tucson's quality-of-life issues. The goal is to leave the Community Forum with a better understanding of key issues that affect the health and quality of life in the community, factors that motivate health, and obstacles that hinder it. The Community Forum also sought consensus regarding priorities, processes, and the next steps for community action.

The Daughters of Charity National Health System The Daughters of Charity National Health System, based in St. Louis, Missouri, is another example of a vision-led system. The Daughters of Charity National Health System's mission, vision, and values statement is reproduced as figure 1-1. The vision of the Daughters of Charity National Health System is based on special concern for the sick and poor and the promotion of a healthy and just society.

Principle 4: Promote Stewardship

The fourth governance principle calls for organizations to choose stewardship over self-interest. A major obstacle in many of our organizations is that, as one board chair told me, "We tend to externalize the problem." Conversations about stewardship seem to turn to the need for other organizations to change or work to solve the health issues facing communities. Some boards feel that if they wait to take action, the city, state, or federal government will deal with community health problems.

This attitude prevents organizations from reaching their full potential. The truth is that health care organizations have the capacity and the capability to deal with all the health issues facing communities. Experts on health exist in every health care organization. They are the board members, physicians, researchers, health educators, managers, epidemiologists, and social workers, to name only a few. Health care organizations already have the human resources and the financial resources to deal effectively with the health issues facing communities. With good intentions and a willingness to become community stewards, these institutions can improve community health.

Stewardship should begin within organizations and extend into the communities they serve. This fourth governance principle promotes the collective exploration, assessment, and design of a healthy community. Broad community participation with others suggests involvement of the business community, not-for-profit organizations, city and state government, the public health department, the local chamber of commerce, the police department, local churches, and the school system.

The Healthier Tucson Community Forum described above is an excellent example of how a sense of stewardship led local leaders representing different community interests to collaborate for the betterment of the community as a whole. Another organization that exemplifies community stewardship is Connecticut Children's Medical Center.

Connecticut Children's Medical Center The board of the Connecticut Children's Medical Center in Hartford, Connecticut, understands that service is central to stewardship. One board member stated to me that

FIGURE 1-1. The Daughters of Charity National Health System's Mission, Vision, and Values

The Daughters of Charity health ministry advances and strengthens the healing mission of the Catholic Church through ideas, influence and actions. We will be faithful to the tradition of service established by St. Vincent de Paul, St. Louise de Marillac and St. Elizabeth Ann Seton.

Our MISSION is to make a positive difference in the lives and health status of individuals and communities. Central to our mission is service to those persons who are poor. The health services we provide will be spiritually-centered, accessible and affordable.

Our VISION is a strong, vibrant Catholic health ministry in the United States in the 21st century. We are committed to partnering with those with whom we share compatible values, including other sponsors, physicians, and associates. We believe the laity are partners in sharing responsibility for the health ministry.

Our vision demands transformation and calls us to:

- advocate a humane and just society, with special concern for those persons who are poor and vulnerable
- emphasize a culture that embraces learning, diversity, collaboration and the well-being of our associates
- strengthen the development of religious and lay leaders
- commit ourselves to all aspects of health—community health, personal health, disease management, and spirituality
- achieve a full continuum of care—a balance of home, community, ambulatory, and inpatient services—to meet preventive, acute, and chronic needs
- foster growth to strengthen the ministry through partnerships, acquisitions, and diversification
- invest in change by demonstrating the value of innovation

We must transform our governance, service models, and thinking to continue our mission and achieve this vision. In keeping with St. Vincent de Paul, "Let us put confidence in our Lord, for He will be with us first and last in the accomplishment of a work to which He has called us."

Our core VALUES inspire our mission, and our vision as the Charity of Christ urges us toward:

Respect, Quality Service, Simplicity, Advocacy for the Poor, and Inventiveness to Infinity.

Source: The Daughters of Charity Health Ministry, Mission, Visions and Values, St. Louis, Mo., Nov. 4, 1996. Printed with permission.

"We must be as busy outside the four walls of our medical center [as inside] and serve the children before they need us." Below are just some of the initiatives they have implemented to serve and improve the health of children:

- *The Children's Fund of Connecticut:* Connecticut Children's Medical Center contributed $15 million to The Children's Fund of Connecticut, which is used to fund innovative community-based primary and preventive health care initiatives in Connecticut. With donations from the corporate community and other health care providers, the fund has grown to $22 million.
- *Teen pregnancy prevention:* The Hartford Action Plan on Infant Health, the City of Hartford Board of Education, the Connecticut Department of Education, Hartford Hospital, St. Francis Hospital, and Connecticut Children's Medical Center founded a teen pregnancy prevention program. Using a professionally prepared curriculum, high school seniors teach fifth graders about reproductive health. The goal of the program is to help shape children's behaviors at an early age.
- *Violence Intervention Project (VIP):* The Hartford Police Department, the Village for Families and Children, the Institute for the Hispanic Family, St. Francis Hospital, the Institute of Living, and the Connecticut Children's Medical Center created the VIP project, whose goal it is to respond quickly to the psychological needs of children who have been witnesses to violence. Police officers call a central number at one of the participating agencies to report an incident in which a child needs immediate on-site response or next-day follow-up and support through a child guidance program at an accessible agency.
- *The Connecticut Childhood Injury Prevention Center:* The Injury Prevention Center houses the Safe Kids Coalition for Connecticut, which is designed to promote bicycle safety for young children. The center is involved in professional education of providers on assessment and intervention with respect to children and teens involved in or witnessing violence, providing legislative testimony, public awareness, and advocacy, and addressing public policy with regard to violence, childhood safety, and teenage suicide prevention.
- *The Manhole Cover Project—A Gun Legacy:* This project is a community-based public art project cosponsored by the Wadsworth Atheneum and The Connecticut Childhood Injury Prevention Center of the Connecticut Children's Medical Center. The Wadsworth held an exhibition of 228 manhole covers made from 39,256 pounds of iron— or the equivalent of the weight of the 11,194 guns confiscated by the Connecticut State Police since 1992—and recorded audio testimonies given by individuals in Hartford whose lives have been profoundly affected by gun violence. The Manhole Cover Project both responds

to the problem of contemporary gun violence in Hartford and acknowledges the role that guns have played in the city's history.

These are just a few of the ways the Connecticut Children's Medical Center Board participates in partnership with others to serve the children and improve their health and well-being for generations to come.

The Carter Center In 1982, former U.S. President Jimmy Carter and his wife Rosalynn founded The Carter Center in Atlanta, Georgia. Their vision of the center is a place where people can come together to resolve their differences and solve problems. The mission statement says, "The Carter Center brings people and resources together to promote peace and human rights, resolve conflicts, foster democracy and development, and fight poverty, hunger, and disease throughout the world." By drawing on the experience and participation of President Carter and other world leaders, by fostering collaboration and avoiding duplication of existing efforts, and by combining effective action plans with research and analysis, the center can achieve goals beyond the reach of single individuals or organizations. The center is guided by the principle that with the necessary skills, knowledge, and access to resources, people can improve their own lives and the lives of others.

Principle 5: Empower the Organization and the Community

The fifth and last governance principle suggests that boards funnel their energy into empowering both their organizations and their communities to create health. This principle calls for organizations to shift from an internal focus to a focus on both the internal and external environments. Equal time is spent at board meetings discussing the success of the organization and the health status of the population served. The board becomes involved with others in the community, listening to their perspectives, facilitating discussion and distribution of resources, and transforming the way health is perceived and delivered. One board chair told me, "We must empower the organization and community to collectively act to improve the health status of the community." The following case examples illustrate this shift in focus.

Hackley Hospital Hackley Hospital in Muskegon, Michigan, moved away from the past by building a stronger connection to neighborhoods. A key element of the board's mission is to build networks in the community as part of a strategy to improve the health status of the community. Health care providers were linked with the neighborhoods to create a health care delivery system that reflects the needs and priorities of the community. By building stronger connections to the community neighborhoods, power was shared equally, and a health care delivery system that better met the health needs of the community was created.

Kalamazoo Healthy Futures Forum Kalamazoo, Michigan, launched the Healthy Futures Initiative in the spring of 1995. Developed by a "leadership cabinet" including the mayors of Kalamazoo and Portage, CEOs of major corporations, clergy, national and state lawmakers, foundation heads, and representatives from the chamber of commerce and local health care systems. The forum gave stakeholders from around the county the opportunity to learn the principles of the healthier communities process and to share the findings of a community assessment conducted by a consulting firm. Despite the generally favorable conclusions in the assessment, stakeholders saw the need for improvement in several areas, including poverty, crime, teenage pregnancy, and domestic violence. In addition, the stakeholders agreed to boost child immunization rates.

As the Kalamazoo Healthy Futures Forum illustrates, *empowerment* means that the organization and the community work together in new ways. By developing a shared vision of health and identifying priorities, both the organization and the community work together to create health.

LESSONS FROM THE FIELD

"Don't let the status quo seduce you. While you're reviewing last year's strategic plan and wearing out the carpet by walking the same old paths, you might miss big opportunities or, worse, put the entire organization in jeopardy. It's tough risking the advantages you've worked so hard to build, but that's one of the prices of leadership."

As is illustrated by the case examples above, many health care organizations have already adopted one or more of the five principles of contemporary governance with notable success. By analyzing their successes, we can more clearly understand what it will take to develop better health care organizations and healthier communities in the future. At the same time, it is equally important to look at initiatives that have failed. In this way, we can learn from the mistakes of others and better understand how to sustain our gains.

Many boards have attempted to apply one or more of the five principles of 21st-century governance only to fall back to their old patterns and ways of doing things. The case examples that follow describe their failed attempts and suggest ways that the failures could have been avoided.

An Attempt to Create the Conditions for a New Order

In attempting to apply the first governance principle—*create the conditions for a new order to emerge*—one board member described a recent board retreat where the trustees "got rid of our old and tired board committees. We tried to create a new environment internally and to externally talk to those who historically had been our competitors. Our new committee structure came out of a new set of board priorities, including issues like affiliation, healthy community, and integration with physicians. Three months after the retreat, I realized nothing would actually change, and it didn't. We fell back to our old ways of doing things."

What went wrong? The affiliation priority in this case led to serious discussions with the competing hospital and several nonacute care providers. A new set of board priorities was supposed to drive the organization in a new direction. The trustees even attempted to open a dialogue with their competitors. But the organization was still too "self-centered" to move ahead; the board went back to maintaining the status quo and protecting the old way of governing.

In this case, this board did not follow through sufficiently. The most powerful thing the governance team can do is initiate and sustain the leadership for community change. The goal is to create the environment that breaks down historical barriers and develops the capacity for new and existing leadership. Broad-based collaborative approaches for addressing community health only succeed if they are sufficiently developed and sustained. The community shares the power, and there are equal players moving forward. The lesson for governance teams is that a board that truly acts on the basis of the first principle of contemporary governance will create the conditions under which a new order will emerge.

An Attempt to Define Health Care in Terms of Community Health

Another board member described her organization's attempt to apply the second principle of 21st-century governance—*redefine health care in terms of disease management and community health:*

> We began to understand the needs of the young people in our community. We had one of the highest teen homicide rates, and we reached out to many of the teens in our community. We set a course and founded a violence intervention initiative. We really focused on a health issue of significance to our community. Teen homicide and violence decreased significantly. We saved young

lives. We reached out, understood the issue, and became stewards of the community. Our mission drove this one simple initiative. The goal wasn't to focus on the hospital anymore. It felt good, it was fun to be on the board, but then we fell back into our old habits.

In this example, the board focused on teen homicide. This organization defined health care in a broad sense, and instead of focusing on taking care of teens in the emergency room after a violent event as the primary intervention, they decided to focus on violence prevention. They focused on keeping teens well and avoiding a course of hospitalization and rehabilitation. After one very successful initiative, however, nothing else came along to keep the fire going. To support and sustain these kinds of initiatives, boards must stay focused on the fundamental issues that create health in the communities they serve.

An Attempt to Become Vision and Mission Driven

In describing her organization's vision to create one health care system in a two-hospital town, a board member said: "We knew we had to redefine our hospital's role in the community. It was a matter of survival. After several unsuccessful attempts, we decided to merge with our sister hospital and create one integrated system of care, ready to compete with others in our region. We didn't succeed. I suppose it became more important, because of a few individuals, to preserve the status quo. We were internally focused."

In this case, being internally focused sabotaged the board's attempt to apply the third principle of 21st-century governance—*become vision and mission driven*. When boards are vision driven, they focus on the longer term and the steps that need to be taken to achieve the vision. The vision is driven by the needs of the community and the organization and never by a few individuals. The lesson for governance teams is that the board's ability to keep its eye on the horizon is fundamental to achieving the vision.

An Attempt to Promote Stewardship

Another trustee shared the time when his health care organization tried to work with business and community organizations to conduct a health status assessment and to set its community health priorities, thus following the fourth governance principle—*promote stewardship*. "We knew collectively we would be better community stewards if we worked together to identify our community's health priorities." Analysis of community perceptions from the health status assessment, in conjunction with health assessment data, revealed the community's most critical health concerns were alcohol and drugs, teenage pregnancy, unintentional injuries, and domestic violence. "After thoughtful consideration of the issues and a good year's worth of work," the trustee remembered, "the community began to fragment. Competing interventions were developed, and the focus became less on the community and more on our individual organizations."

The health care organization in this example collaborated with others, conducted a health status assessment, and identified its community's most critical health concerns. Clearly there was a well-intentioned effort to collectively design and empower the participants to improve the health of the community. But eventually the focus became internal and "more on our individual organizations." Self-interest overtook stewardship, and competing interventions developed. The lesson for governance teams is that collaborators must come to the design table as equals, commit to stewardship, set aside individual concerns, and work together for the greater good.

An Attempt to Empower the Organization and the Community

Another trustee shared his experiences with a failed attempt to empower the community. A competing health care system from the same area held a forum to discuss and identify community health issues. "Because of the competition between our two systems, only half of the stakeholders were invited to participate in this day-long community forum. My health care system was excluded as were other important players, including the local public health department. How could our community possibly work through its health care issues without all the stakeholders involved? The result was another report, another forum, and another false start."

This initiative obviously failed because only certain segments of the community and selected organizations were invited to participate in the day-long community forum. Underlying the fifth principle of 21st-century governance—*empower the organization and the community*—is the concept of inclusiveness. The only meaningful way to empower the community and other organizations is to bring all the key stakeholders to the table. More often than not, these stakeholders will represent competing interests. It is easy for boards to make decisions based on a path of least resistance or on individual board member concerns. However, decisions must be rooted in a more comprehensive concept of health.

THE RETREAT AS A FORUM FOR CREATING A VISION

"During the retreat, we began to understand our real purpose, and our vision became clear. It was as though somebody hit us over the head with a pound of wisdom. We realized the importance of making decisions based on a belief system. It was a moving experience."

The five principles of 21st-century governance provide a useful framework for transforming governance. However, boards planning to apply the principles may reasonably wonder, Where do we begin? How can we get from where we are today to where we need to be in the future? How do we transform what we do in the boardroom? The single most important approach to transforming what is done in the boardroom is to create a new vision. That is how 21st-century governance teams will effectively make the transition.

Peter Senge, speaking of the importance of a shared vision in *The Fifth Discipline*, states: "If any one idea about leadership has inspired organizations for thousands of years, it's the capacity to hold a shared picture of the future we seek to create. One is hard pressed to think of any organization that has sustained some measure of greatness in the absence of goals, values, and missions that become deeply shared throughout the organization." He goes on to state that "when there is a genuine vision (as opposed to the all-too-familiar 'vision statement'), people excel and learn, not because they are told to, but because they want to."[6]

A clear picture of the future is the first and most important step in making the transition to governance team stewardship. In many cases, the process the board follows to create the vision is just as important as the vision itself.

The Traditional Board Retreat

Most health care organizations create a vision of the future through a retreat process. The traditional board retreat process is primarily driven by internal players and based on 20th-century governance principles. A typical retreat agenda is outlined in figure 1-2.

Traditional retreats can be very effective and lead to lasting results. However, many of the organizations that have embraced the five principles of contemporary governance have taken another approach to creating the vision. With this approach, the community's leadership and, sometimes, whole communities are involved in designing the vision.

FIGURE 1-2. Sample Traditional Retreat Agenda

Day 1

9:30 A.M.-12:00 P.M.
- Introduction, purpose, and approach
- Strategic issues and concerns
- Situation appraisal: an external look
- Situation appraisal: an internal look
- Identification of strategic issues

12:00 P.M.-1:00 P.M.
Lunch

1:00 P.M.-5:00 P.M.
- Group work on the strategic issues
- Report back and discussions of group findings
- Develop options and directions as appropriate
- Summary of the day
- Questions to ponder

Day 2

8:00 A.M.-12:00 P.M.
- Reflection on day 1
- Setting directions
- Clarifying directions
- Next steps
- Action plan
- Adjourn

The Collaborative Retreat

The collaborative retreat includes the trustees of one or more health care organizations plus key stakeholders from the community. Typically, the goal of the retreat is to launch a community future search, that is, a collective agenda for the achievement of community health. Health care organizations that go on a community future search retreat discuss a broad range of issues. Figure 1-3 illustrates a generic future search agenda to create a collaborative community.

Together, participants create a collective vision, written in the present tense. In addition, they set a collaborative community action plan to achieve the vision.

A successful community future search process results in several tangible results. First, the past and present are reviewed and consensus around the community's assets and liabilities or strengths and weaknesses are established. Second, images of future potential or smaller visions are discussed, and these eventually come together to create a

FIGURE 1-3. Sample Collaborative Retreat Agenda

Day 1

9:30 A.M.-12:00 P.M.
- Public interviews with community planners about conference goals
- "Who We Are": introductions and expectations
- Overview of work plan
  - The past: review community history
  - The present: what about community life makes us proudest? Makes us sorriest?
- Consensus priorities
- The future: images of potential
- Desired futures one year from now

12:00 P.M.-2:00 P.M.
Buffet lunch; stakeholders read priorities on images lists

2:00 P.M.-4:00 P.M.
- Select community priorities
- Self-select action groups
- Goals, initial action plans
- Process review—"Pulse taking"

Day 2

9:30 A.M.-12:00 P.M.
- Testing feasibility
- Role-playing skill practice (for example, managing resistance to ideas)

12:00 P.M.-1:30 P.M.
Buffet lunch; community leaders comment on plans

1:30 P.M.-3:30 P.M.
- Follow-up planning: who, what, when
- Task force reports
- Schedule review meeting
- Documentation plans, media interviews

more important vision. The third tangible result is that community priorities are set, typically based on the results of a population-based health status assessment, a tool that aids the community in better understanding the health of the population and in making informed decisions about future investments that will improve the health status of the community. Typically, the assessment consists of an inventory of existing resources, the population's health status, strengths and weaknesses of the current system, and a set of action-based priorities. A fourth tangible result of the collaborative retreat is that goals, an action plan, and assignment of responsibilities are achieved as a result of the collaborative community retreat. The collaborative community retreat is done within the context of the community future search. Board and community leadership participate in the preparation of the agenda, the retreat process, and the expected outcomes. The Kalamazoo Healthy Futures Forum, described previously, is a good example of a community future search.

CONCLUSION

Boards that are committed to and active in creating healthier communities are well on the path to visionary leadership. They adopt the five principles of contemporary governance and believe that creating the conditions under which a new order will emerge is one of their primary roles. Under this type of board, collaboration replaces competition.

In the future, boards will broaden their definition of health, a step that will lead to community stewardship. Community stewardship, in turn, will lead to the collective design of collaborative communities. This emerging model of collaboration will lead to healthier populations, shared community visions, and empowered communities.

References

1. John Carver, *Boards That Make A Difference: A New Design for Leadership in Nonprofit and Public Organizations* (San Francisco: Jossey-Bass, 1990), pp. xii–xiii. Reprinted with permission.

2. Peter Block, *Stewardship: Choosing Service over Self-Interest* (San Francisco: Berrett-Koehler, 1993), p. 6.

3. Greater Manchester Chamber of Commerce. *The Manchester Agenda* (Manchester, N.H., 1993).

4. Memorial Hospital and Health System of South Bend, *Creating a Healthy Community* (South Bend, Ind., 1994), pp. 5–6. Used with permission.

5. Northwest Community Healthcare, *Mission/Vision/Values and Guiding Principles* (Arlington Heights, Ill., 1997), p. 1. Used with permission.

6. Peter Senge, *The Fifth Discipline: The Art and Practice of the Learning Organization* (New York: Doubleday/Currency, 1990), p. 9.

2

Taking the Path to the Healthy Community

The significant problems we face cannot be solved at the same level of thinking we were at when we created them.

—*Albert Einstein*

A s we move into the 21st century, the development of healthy communities has taken on a new importance. For both economic and altruistic reasons, boards and their health care organizations are taking a more active role in promoting the overall health and welfare of their communities.

The notion of a healthy community is, of course, not new. The World Health Organization (WHO) introduced the healthy cities/community concept at an international conference more than 10 years ago. The idea began with a feasibility study in 1985 and was further developed at an international conference of the WHO in Ottawa, Ontario, in 1986. By 1992, more than 400 cities worldwide had joined the healthy cities movement.[1] According to the WHO, "The healthy cities project challenges cities to take seriously the process of developing health-enhancing public policies that create physical and social environments that support health, and strengthen community action for health."[2] Today, more than 2,000 healthy community initiatives are in various stages of development worldwide. The challenge for our own health care organizations is to take seriously the process of developing health in our own communities and to strengthen community involvement.

But what is health, and what role do our boards and organizations play in creating it? How should they relate to others in the community? How do they enlist the aid of others and gain their support? This chapter presents several authoritative definitions of community health, looks at the importance of collaboration in creating it, and examines three paths that boards can take to build health in their own communities.

DEFINITIONS OF A HEALTHY COMMUNITY

"The board as an entity maintains a balance between institutional and community values."

Before embarking on the journey to a healthy community, boards should have a clear understanding of what a healthy community is. By looking at several definitions of community health, boards can create signposts to guide themselves on their own journeys.

Hancock and Duhl's Definition

T. Hancock and L. Duhl define a healthy city as "one that is continually creating and improving those physical and social environments and expanding those community resources which enable people to mutually support each other in performing all the functions of life and in developing to their maximum potential."[3] They go on to define a set of qualities a city should strive to provide. (See figure 2-1.)

It is reasonable to ask whether such qualities as adequate housing, a stable ecosystem, and a vital economy are within the scope of what trustees do in health care and within the purview of governance. The answer is that a broader definition of health demands no less. The qualities of a healthy city are a good starting point for governance teams to understand what health is and how it might be measured.

In response to the new emphasis on community health, several organizations have developed definitions of a healthy community. They include Memorial Hospital and Health System, Inc., of South Bend, Indiana, the National Civic League, and the U.S. Public Health Service.

The Memorial Hospital and Health System's Definition

The Memorial Hospital and Health System, Inc., of South Bend, Indiana, states, "There are two very important ingredients you'll need if you're going to create a healthier community. First, you'll need to define health. Next you'll need to define your community." Memorial's definition of a healthy community is as follows:

Healthy communities actively work to improve the health and quality of life of all their residents. Therefore, the definition of health goes beyond the absence of disease and the traditional medical concept and addresses the underlying factors in quality of life, such as the environment, crime, and literacy.

In this context, a healthy community is one in which everyone has the opportunity to

FIGURE 2-1. The Qualities of a Healthy City

The Qualities of a Healthy City

A city should strive to provide:

1. a clean, safe and physical environment of high quality (including housing quality)
2. an ecosystem that is stable now and sustainable in the long term
3. a strong, mutually supportive and nonexploitative community
4. a high degree of participation and control by the public over the decisions affecting their lives, health, and well-being
5. the meeting of basic needs (for food, water, shelter, income safety, and work) for all the city's people
6. access to a wide variety of experiences and resources, with the chance for a wide variety of contact, interaction, and communication
7. a diverse, vital, and innovative city economy
8. the encouragement of connectiveness with the past, with the cultural and biological heritage of city dwellers and with other groups and individuals
9. a form that is compatible with and enhances the preceding characteristics
10. an optimum level of appropriate public health and sick care services accessible to all
11. high health status (high levels of positive health and low levels of disease)

Source: T. Hancock and L. Duhl, *Promoting Health in the Urban Context,* WHO Healthy Cities Paper No. 1 (Copenhagen: FADL, 1988).

- access and receive high quality, affordable medical care
- exercise preventive health practice
- breathe clean air
- drink clean water
- live in adequate housing
- learn to the extent of their capacity and desire
- experience artistic stimuli
- worship in the religion of their choosing
- find rewarding recreational activities
- work in a safe environment
- be safe from bodily harm

To achieve and maintain this optimal healthy community, a myriad of forces must work together. Some of these forces include, but are not limited to, area governmental agencies, educational institutions, arts organizations, health care providers, criminal justice agencies, chambers of commerce, insurance providers, employers, and media providers.[4]

Many of the qualities described in Memorial's definition of a healthy community parallel those outlined by Hancock and Duhl. Both definitions stress the importance of the factors that contribute to the quality of life, including a clean, safe, and wholesome environment.

The National Civic League's Definition

Another organization that advocates a civic agenda to create healthy communities that work for everyone is the National Civic League. This organization promotes the involvement of citizens in the governance of their communities. The National Civic League encourages citizen participation, collaborative problem solving, conscience-based decision making, and diversity.

In defining what constitutes healthy communities, the National Civic League cites the qualities developed by the WHO:

> Healthy Communities work with a broad definition of health that goes beyond the absence of disease to address the underlying factors that create health and a high quality of life. A healthy community, according to the World Health Organization, includes characteristics such as a clean, safe, high quality physical environment and a sustainable ecosystem; the provision of basic needs; an optimum level of appropriate, high quality, accessible public health and sick care services; quality educational opportunity; and a diverse, vital and innovative economy. In healthy communities, health-related outcomes are effectively addressed through broad based community involvement. The focus is on the total community—social, economic, geographic, and political—as the ideal context for health promotion. Private citizens and the business, nonprofit, and governmental sectors work cooperatively to define a desired future, clarify the issues and implement innovative solutions.[5]

The U.S. Public Health Service's Definition

The U.S. Public Health Service offers a flexible definition:

> The single defining feature of a Healthy City or Community is that its citizens, in all their various roles, have joined forces to pursue positive change. No matter who initiates the Healthy City/

Community process, that initiator brings all the other players into the game. Healthy City and Community project participants recognize the power of localities to make significant positive changes in the health of their citizens. The movement is based on a philosophy that places equal emphasis on the process of promoting change as well as the ultimate consequences of that process. Among Healthy Cities projects, process and outcomes are inextricably linked. As a result, there can be no single model for a Healthy City or Community. Each community is unique in the problems it faces and in the resources, cultures, infrastructure, and approaches it takes to respond to those problems.[6]

Healthy People 2000

Healthy People 2000 is another initiative to improve the health of all Americans through prevention. It is driven by 300 specific national health promotion and disease prevention objectives targeted for achievement by the year 2000. Healthy People 2000's overall goals are to

- increase the span of healthy life for Americans
- reduce health disparities among Americans
- achieve access to preventive services for all Americans[7]

While the initiatives all underline different priorities and values, they share some important characteristics:

- Their definition of health includes overall well-being and quality of life.
- They advocate a community-wide approach to identifying priorities and developing and implementing plans.
- They understand the value of structural change at the local level to the real improvement in community well-being.

Every kind of health care organization now aims to build healthy communities, and governance teams are an integral part of these efforts. Twenty-first-century governance will adopt a new definition of health that will result in greater collaboration and a new and more important vision for our health care organizations.

THE TRANSITION FROM COMPETITION TO COLLABORATION

"We must develop the concept of shared community governance, collaborate, and create strategic alliances in ways we never have in the past . . . We must make decisions based on a new set of principles."

Health care at the end of the 20th century is characterized by competition. As pointed out in chapter 1, the tendency in health care governance has been to focus on the needs of the organization. In this competitive environment, money and power are preeminent, and organizations try to gain market share at the expense of other organizations. In contrast, 21st-century governance will be characterized by collaboration. The new emphasis on creating healthier communities will impel boards and their organizations to collaborate with other community leaders to increase their ability to create health.

Definition of Collaboration

According to Arthur T. Himmelman, collaboration consists of "exchanging information, altering activities, sharing resources, and enhancing capacity of another for mutual benefit and to achieve a common purpose." He continues, "When considering collaboration as a change strategy, it can be useful to view it in relationship to three other common change strategies—networking, coordination and cooperation—that can be defined as building upon each other along a continuum of complexity and commitment. Each of these four strategies can be appropriate for particular circumstances depending on levels of trust and the degree to which there are a common vision, commitments to share power, and responsible and accountable actions."

Himmelman's definitions for networking, coordination, and cooperation are as follows:

- *Networking:* "Exchanging information for mutual benefit."
- *Coordinating:* "Exchanging information and altering activities for mutual benefit and to achieve a common purpose."
- *Cooperation:* "Exchanging information, altering activities, and sharing resources for mutual benefit and to achieve a common purpose."[8]

True collaboration occurs when networking, coordination, and cooperation are all used in conjunction with each other. It is possible to build collaborative organizations as well as collaborative communities. Both can develop around a common vision that enhances the capacity of the organization and the community to achieve health in the community.

Three Organizational Stages on the Path to Collaboration

During the 21st century, governance teams will recognize that the only means to achieving a broader vision is through true collaboration with many different sectors of the community. They will identify the various stakeholders in the community and encourage cooperation and collaboration. As organizations make the transition from competition to collaboration, they move through three distinct stages. (See table 2-1.)

Stage I Organizations Stage I organizations concentrate primarily on internal improvement processes. A collaborative environment is created, but collaboration consists of internal teams working in concert to improve both the quality of care and the quality of the business practice. Governance information is more limited during stage I, and health care is viewed from a narrow definition—a 20th-century definition of health, with its focus on eliminating disease. The focus on sick care leads stage I organizations to concentrate on admissions, procedures, and encounters. During this stage, significant clinical gains are made and quality is enhanced, but again, these achievements are internal.

Stage II Organizations As organizations move closer to collaboration, they enter stage II, which is marked by a shift in focus to the community and the well-being of the population. In these organizations, the governance team begins to act from 21st-century governance principles, and community improvement begins to take precedence over the individual organization's needs. Because health care is defined in terms of disease management and community health, the organization seeks the assistance of institutions and agencies in the community. The organization now becomes both vision- and mission-driven and moves visibly from self-interest to promoting stewardship. Service becomes the priority, and the profits follow. The health of the population becomes paramount, regardless of the site of care or who is delivering the care.

Northwest Community Healthcare in Arlington Heights, Illinois, is a stage II organization. Its commitment to community is reflected in its mission statement, which is quoted in chapter 1, and in its vision and action statements, which are reproduced in figure 2-2.

TABLE 2-1. From Competition to Collaboration

Competition ⟶			Collaboration
1980s	Mid- to late 1990s	Year 2000 to 2010	21st Century
	(Stage I)	(Stage II)	(Stage III)
Market-driven competition	Organization improvement process	Community improvement process	Global improvement process

FIGURE 2-2. Vision Statement, Northwest Community Healthcare

Vision—By the year 2000, we will be the preeminent health partner for the northwest community.

As the preeminent healthcare partner it is our responsibility to create a healthier community by improving the health and well-being of all community members through education and prevention.

Ideally, our prevention efforts are so successful that the measured health of our community improves from year to year. Should there be health problems, it is our responsibility to ensure that community members receive quality care in the least expensive setting with the best possible outcome.

It is also our responsibility to ensure that the delivery of care focuses on the needs of the total person, so that quality of life and dignity are maintained. Patient-centered care requires changing the goals of clinical care in order to meet the needs and expectations of the patient. Patients measure quality of care by what effect, good or bad, it has on their lives. Looking at the patient as a whole person rather than as a diagnosis is key to gauging patient outcomes.

This vision requires us to see ourselves as not just a hospital, but as a series of settings including hospitals, physician offices, nursing homes, home health care, day surgery centers, day care centers, and fitness centers that function as a system.

To realize this vision will require collaborative partnerships among all sectors of the community and tremendous coordination of services within the Northwest Community Healthcare System.

Source: Northwest Community Healthcare, *Mission/Vision/Values and Guiding Principles* (Arlington Heights, Ill., 1997), p. 1. Used with permission.

Stage III Organizations Finally, as we improve the health status of our own communities, the collective wisdom will shift to more global issues, which represent a transition to stage III. Stage III organizations will focus on such issues as the environment, health status of defined populations, education, diversity, the economy, and quality of life. Regions, states, and nations will be called to action by regional, state, and national initiatives. National initiatives and priorities will take on greater significance as nations come together to improve health globally. Stage III represents a mature, healthy community movement for all society. Our civilization will enter stage III sometime beyond the year 2010.

Key Characteristics of Collaborative Organizations

As governance teams and their organizations move through the three stages, they will display four key characteristics that emerge from 21st-century governance principles. These characteristics may be viewed as guideposts on the path to healthier communities:

- a commitment to a broad community health vision
- the alignment of the interests of the community and the organization
- collaboration with others and the development of partnerships
- a balance between autonomy and dependency

When health is defined more broadly, then the vision is broad. Boards on the cusp of stage II will know immediately, because they will redefine who they are, what they stand for, and how they behave. They will establish a new kind of relationship with the community, and over time their organizations will develop into preeminent health partners. The boards will begin to understand that a shared vision results in the alignment of the community's and the organization's interests and in the achievement of mutual goals. Collaboration will be a matter of necessity, and autonomy will be balanced by interdependency.

A Model of Participation

An alternative model of the transition from competition to collaboration is offered by Sherry R. Arnstein. She envisions the process as a climb up a staircase of citizen participation. (See figure 2-3.) The first five steps of the staircase characterize the organization's relationship with the community as one of nonparticipation and tokenism. These first five steps resemble stage I organizations described above. The health care organization's interaction with the community is passive, and in some cases it may even be manipulative if the organization is using the community as a means to an end. The quality of interaction improves further up the staircase.

The top three steps resemble stage II organizations. As the community assumes more equality in the collaboration, the provider moves closer to a true partnership in which power is shared. Only if there is equality will the community say that the health care organization is truly its partner.

Without the equality necessary to deal with other organizations and other people, healthy communities will not come into existence. Governance teams that have created stage II organizations will actually hold discussions on community relations and use phrases like "broader vision," "collaborative community," "alignment of interests," and "the need to balance autonomy with dependency." As the health care paradigm moves from competition to collaboration, collaborative communities will focus on improving the health of the population.

FIGURE 2-3. The Staircase of Citizen Participation

Partnership
Community groups that
are empowered in an
equal relationship with
"power-holding"
organizations

Shared Power

Delegated Power
Majority of decision-making
seats to "non-power-holders"

Citizen Control
Decision-making clout entirely
in hand of non-power-holders

Informing
Providers educate the
community

Consultation
Providers consult community
on actions/issues without
ensuring views will be heeded

Tokenism

Placation
Interaction primarily directed at
avoiding community revolt

Manipulation
Educate community to support
end of the organization

Therapy
Interact with the community as
if it is passive; attempt to "cure"
without active involvement of
those they are trying to cure

Nonparticipation

Source: VHA, Inc., *Community Partnerships: Taking Charge of Change Through Partnership* (Irving, Tex.: VHA, Inc., 1993), p. 35. Adapted from S. R. Arnstein, "A Ladder of Citizen Participation," *AIP Journal* (July 1969): 216–24. Used with permission.

FRAMEWORKS FOR CREATING HEALTHY COMMUNITIES

"The real board lesson came when there was a change in our mental model, a departure from the 'brick and mortar' attitude toward one focused on improving the health of the community. Health cannot be defined by the hospital, but must be defined by the community."

In the past, health care organizations have been challenged to formulate strategies to achieve accountability within the community. As a result, several frameworks have been developed to assist governance teams to move forward with initiatives that improve the health status of a geographic population. These frameworks begin to move us closer to the 21st-century governance principles. Many health care organizations and their governance teams began their healthy community initiatives using such frameworks. The three frameworks include the Hospital Community Benefit Standards Program, the VHA's Voluntary Community Benefits Standards, and the Catholic Health Association's Standards for Community Benefit.

The Hospital Community Benefits Standards Program

The Hospital Community Benefits Standards Program was a national demonstration initiative funded by the W. K. Kellogg Foundation and administered by the Robert F. Wagner Graduate School of Public Health at New York University. In 1989, a National Steering Committee developed four standards for hospital community benefit programs. (See appendix 2-1 at the end of this chapter.)

Standard 1: Committing to a Community Benefit Program To meet the first standard, hospitals had to show evidence of a formal commitment to a community benefit program for a designated community. Many of the 49 health care organizations that participated in the demonstration project did so through newly revised visions that included a statement about community benefit. Governance teams also showed evidence of commitment through projects that improved the health status of their community. In addition, boards formally authorized their CEOs to conduct and oversee all activities related to the Hospital Community Benefits Program and approved the goals, objectives, and a plan of operation for the community benefit program. This approach lent structure to the launch of the healthy community process.

Standard 2: Sponsoring Community Projects The second standard called for hospital-sponsored community projects for improving health status, focusing on (1) addressing the health problems of minorities, the poor, and other medically underserved populations, and (2) containing the growth of community health care costs. In response to standard 2, health care organizations sponsored a number of projects, including:

- development of prenatal care programs with a goal to increase access and improve the birth weights of high-risk babies
- development of free care policies

- development of primary care school-based programs
- development of a community health center
- investigation of the feasibility of sharing high technology with other health care organizations
- assessment of the health care needs of low-income children and of the feasibility of delivering primary care through satellite programs

Governance teams provided funding for projects that improved the health of the community. In some instances, the governance teams funded existing providers so that they could expand their capacity to deliver health care services that were lacking.

Standard 3: Enlisting Other Organizations The third standard called for hospitals to launch activities designed to stimulate other organizations and individuals to join in carrying out a broad health agenda in the designated community. As a result of this standard, many of the health care organizations in the demonstration project developed close working relationships with local businesses, industries, and the chamber of commerce; local churches and schools; state, city, and town governments; and community organizations. They also noted the importance of the role of public health and the public health department. Public health focuses on preventive measures and programs of immunization, water quality, sanitation, and safety, to name just a few. In short, public health focuses on measures that society can take to ensure that people live under healthy conditions. The governance teams of organizations that met this third standard repeatedly stated that the success of their efforts depended on their ability to enlist others to join in carrying out a broad health agenda.

Standard 4: Fostering a Positive Internal Environment The last standard required hospitals to foster an internal environment that encouraged organization-wide involvement in the program. For many of the hospitals in the demonstration project, meeting this standard meant sharing the broader vision in a town meeting format and at medical staff meetings. Organizations also encouraged broad participation by involving medical staff, employees, and volunteers in such activities as working at the local soup kitchen, sponsoring a coat drive, or assisting a family over the holidays.

It is interesting to note that the single most important factor in enlisting organization-wide participation was the support of the governing body. In each instance, the governing body designated the community as the focus of the hospital's program, adopted a revised vision statement, and committed to carry out the program. Many of the organizations provided their governance teams with facts and figures about community problems, such as the number of people underserved, patterns of teen drug use in the community, and the health care needs of low-income children in the school system. Many in this national demonstration project learned that board support and involvement early on is critical to implementing a community health agenda. For many governance teams, this framework created the structure to move forward and to begin the healthy community process.

VHA's Voluntary Community Benefits Standards

A second framework for creating healthier communities is VHA's Voluntary Community Benefits Standards: A Framework for Meeting Community Health Needs. Within this framework, five standards were developed. (See figure 2-4.)

> Standard 1. demonstrate leadership as a charitable institution
> Standard 2. provide essential healthcare services
> Standard 3. be accountable to the community
> Standard 4. evidence commitment to community benefit
> Standard 5. operate free from private profit[9]

Governance teams of VHA hospitals across the country adopted this framework for meeting community health needs. Early board commitment to these standards was also critical to moving forward. Following are some examples of VHA organizations that adopted these standards.

U.S. Health Corporation The U.S. Health Corporation in Columbus, Ohio, participates in the Franklin County Leadership Council to reduce infant mortality. The council consists of more than 100 members, among them county leaders and such health care professionals as physicians, hospital administrators, and nurse practitioners. Organizations include hospitals; insurance companies; city, county, and state governments; trade associations; professional societies; child welfare agencies; the United Way; the Columbus Area Chamber of Commerce; the Columbus Foundation; the Columbus Board of Education; and Ohio State University. The goal of the council is to establish a countywide collaborative action to bring the infant mortality rate of Franklin County in line with the nation's goal of 7 per 1,000 live births by or before the year 2000.

Hartford Hospital Hartford Hospital in Hartford, Connecticut, is a key member of the Hartford Action Plan on Infant Health, a partnership of public and private sectors working to reduce infant mortality and teen pregnancy in Hartford. The Hartford Action Plan brings together major

FIGURE 2-4. VHA's Voluntary Community Benefits Standards

Standard #1: Demonstrate leadership as a charitable institution

Minimum guidelines:

- Assert leadership in organizing community-wide efforts for the needy
- Reach out to the underserved to provide needed primary and preventive health care services and health education
- Attract and use donated funds to serve the needy
- Participate in Medicaid and other federal, state and local health care reimbursement programs for the needy
- Formally plan for and provide charity care or maintain an open door policy to the extent of financial ability

Standard #2: Provide essential health care services

Minimum guidelines:

- Cooperate with other community health care providers to maximize the meeting of essential community health needs
- Render health care services and educational services that are specifically designed to meet assessed community needs and improve community health status
- Operate a 24-hour emergency room to the extent needed by the community

Standard #3: Be accountable to the community

Minimum guidelines:

- Have a volunteer governing board composed of members of the community the hospital serves
- Invite and respond to community input and involvement in the planning and review of hospital activities
- Voluntarily disclose information on hospital services, financial status, community benefit activities and charity care to the public
- Advocate health care cost containment efforts and promote the efficient use of health care resources within the community

Standard #4: Evidence commitment to community benefit

Minimum guidelines:

- Embrace a mission statement and bylaws that reflect a commitment to a charitable purpose and community benefit
- Provide leadership for organizing community-wide efforts for enhancing community health

FIGURE 2-4. *(Continued)*

- Integrate a community benefits plan based on assessments of community health needs into overall strategic plan
- Educate and involve employees and medical staff in the provision of community benefits

Standard #5: Operate free from private profit

Minimum guidelines:

- Maintain a corporate and legal structure that meets all requirements for not-for-profit status
- Ensure that affiliated business enterprises serve the hospital's charitable purpose and present no conflicts of interest with the not-for-profit, charitable mission of the hospital
- Employ financial surpluses to further the institution's charitable purpose and not to promote private inurement to any individual

---

Source: VHA, Inc., *Community Partnerships: Taking Charge of Change Through Partnership* (Irving, Tex.: VHA, Inc., 1993), p. 3. Used with permission.

health care providers, businesses, schools, city and state governments, and community organizations. The plan is guided by a shared vision of Hartford as a city where "every young person is self-sufficient before becoming a parent and every baby is born healthy and at full term."

St. Luke's Methodist Hospital In 1989, St. Luke's Methodist Hospital in Cedar Rapids, Iowa, collaborated with key community leaders to develop the nation's first rural model for a child protection center. The center saves the lives of nearly 1,000 children per year. St. Luke's also formed community-directed programs for low-income clients, and with the cooperation of a local community college, created a health and learning center in a rural hospital. Yet another partnership is the Five Season Day Care Center, which offers infant care, before- and after-school programs, and at-risk programs. The center, which was developed in conjunction with a local school district, is now the largest provider of not-for-profit day care in the state.[10]

The Catholic Health Association Standards for Community Benefit

A third framework for creating healthier communities is the Catholic Health Association Standards for Community Benefit. (See figure 2-5.) These standards contain two key elements: (1) the organization's mission and vision statements reflect a future commitment to healthy

FIGURE 2-5. Catholic Health Association Standards for Community Benefit

As members of the Catholic Health Association of the United States, we share a historical mission and tradition of community service. In order to continue our tradition of providing benefit to the community, we affirm that:

1. The organization's mission statements and philosophy should reflect a commitment to benefit the community, and the policies and practices should be consistent with these documents, including:

    -   consideration of operational and policy decisions in light of their impact on the community served, especially the poor, the frail elderly, and the vulnerable.
    -   adoption of charity care policies that are made public and are consistently applied.
    -   incorporation of community healthcare needs into regular planning and budgeting processes.

2. The governing body should adopt, make public, and implement a community benefit plan that:

    -   defines the organization's mission and the community being served.
    -   identifies unmet healthcare needs in the community, including needs of the poor, frail elderly, minorities and other medically underserved and disadvantaged persons.
    -   describes how the organization intends to take a leadership role in advocating community-wide responses to healthcare needs in the community.
    -   describes how the organization intends to address, directly and in collaboration with physicians, other individuals and organizations:
        —particular or unique healthcare problems of the community
        —healthcare needs of the poor, the frail elderly, minorities, and other medically underserved and disadvantaged persons.
    -   describes how the organization sought the views of the community being served and how community members and other organizations were involved in identifying needs and the development of the plan.

FIGURE 2-5. *(Continued)*

3. The healthcare organization should provide community benefits to the poor and the broader community that are designed to:

   • comply with the community benefit plan.
   • improve health status in the community.
   • promote access to healthcare services to all persons in the community.
   • contain healthcare costs.

4. The organization should make available to the public an annual community benefit report that describes the scope of community benefits provided directly and in collaboration with others.

Source: The Catholic Health Association of the United States, *Catholic Health Association Standards for Community Benefit* (Washington, D.C.: CHA, 1992). Used with permission.

communities, and (2) the governing body adopts, makes public, and implements a community benefit plan. The governing body commitment proved to be the starting point. Some examples of Catholic Health Association health care organizations and their accomplishments are described below.

Sacred Heart Health Systems Sacred Heart Health Systems in Eugene, Oregon, has established a close working relationship with Lane County's Health and Human Services Department, community groups, and voluntary agencies to help address some of Eugene's key health care needs. Working with these community groups, Sacred Heart has contributed funds, staff, and facilities, and has won philanthropic support for programs that improve access to prenatal care services for economically disadvantaged women and treatment for substance abuse.

California Pilot Program In 1994, four competing California health care organizations—Mercy Medical Center, Sutter Health, Kaiser Permanente, and the University of California-Davis—collaborated to form a three-year, $1.6 million pilot program. The goal of the program is to improve the health and well-being of the residents of Meadowview, an impoverished section of Sacramento.

CONCLUSION

A new spirit is needed in health care, a spirit embodying the creation and implementation of healthy community agendas. Competition does not fit in with the spirit. Instead, collaboration between health care leaders and other community leaders is required.

Once a definition of community health is agreed on, the transition from a competitive model to a collaborative one can be begun by sharing information, coordinating with others, and working toward a common purpose. The three frameworks described in this chapter suggest ways to initiate action and gain support for creating healthy communities. Thoughtful and determined use of these frameworks can help a board to bring its health care organization into the 21st century, and the 21st-century governance principles can help to keep it on course.

References

1. *Public Policy for Healthy Cities: Involving the Policy Maker, Inaugural Conference of the World Health Organization Collaboration Center in Healthy Cities* (Indianapolis: Institute of Action Research for Community Health, 1992), p. 1.

2. *Public Policy for Healthy Cities*, p. 17.

3. T. Hancock and L. Duhl, *Promoting Health in the Urban Context*, WHO Healthy Cities Paper No. 1 (Copenhagen: FADL, 1988).

4. Memorial Hospital and Health System, Inc., of South Bend, *Creating a Healthy Community* (South Bend, Ind.: Memorial, 1994), pp. 5–6. Used with permission.

5. National Civic League, *Healthy Communities Action Project* (Denver: National Civic League, 1995), p. 2.

6. U.S. Public Health Service, *Starting Points for Creating a Healthy Community* (Washington, D.C.: U.S. Public Health Service, Department of Health and Human Services, 1994), pp. 1–2.

7. U.S. Department of Health and Human Services, Office of Disease Prevention and Health Promotion, *Healthy People 2000* (Washington, D.C.: DHHS, 1991).

8. Arthur T. Himmelman, *Communities Working Collaboratively for a Change* (Minneapolis: Himmelman Consulting Group, 1992), pp. 1–2.

9. VHA, Inc., *Community Partnerships: Taking Charge of Change Through Partnership* (Irving, Tex.: VHA, Inc., 1993), p. 3.

10. *Community Partnerships*, p. 3.

APPENDIX 2-1. Hospital Community Benefits Standards

Standard CB.1 There is evidence of the hospital's formal commitment to a community benefit program for a designated community. *

Required characteristics:

CB.1.1 The governing body is responsible for designating a community as the focus of the hospital's program.
CB.1.2 The governing body adopts a mission statement that includes a commitment to carry out the program.
CB.1.3 The governing body establishes goals and objectives, and approves an operating plan to enable the hospital to:
CB.1.3.1 Carry out projects to improve community health status; address the health problems of minorities, the poor and other medically underserved populations; and contain the growth of community healthcare costs. (See CB.2);
CB.1.3.2 Stimulate other organizations and individuals to join in carrying out a broad community health agenda (see CB.3); and
CB.1.3.3 Foster an internal environment that encourages hospital-wide involvement in the program (see CB.4).
CB.1.4 The community benefit program is effectively managed and regularly evaluated.
CB.1.4.1. The governing body delegates to the chief executive officer the responsibility for overall management of the program.
CB.1.4.2 The chief executive officer or designate carries out managerial tasks including: development of program goals and objectives, program planning, liaison and outreach activities, development of data and information, and day-to-day monitoring and control.
CB.1.4.3 There are mechanisms established to evaluate the program's effectiveness and appropriateness on at least an annual basis.
CB.1.5 There are hospital resources identified to carry out the program activities.
CB.1.6 The hospital participates in the preparation and dissemination of an annual program report which includes:
CB.1.6.1 A disclosure of relevant community-wide data including information on health status; the social problems of minorities, the poor and other medically underserved populations; and healthcare costs of the community.
CB1.6.2 A description of hospital-sponsored projects.

*In these standards, "community" is defined as all persons and organizations within a reasonably circumscribed geographic area, in which there is a sense of interdependence and belonging. Although the singular form of "community" is used, a hospital may designate two or more communities to be part of its community benefit program, as appropriate.

APPENDIX 2-1. *(Continued)*

CB.1.6.3 A description of the hospital's activities that further a broad community health agenda.
CB.1.6.4 An evaluation of the program activities and their respective contributions in achieving program goals and objectives.
CB.1.7 The hospital provides a means for annual public comment on the program's overall effectiveness and appropriateness.

Standard CB.2. The scope of the program includes hospital-sponsored projects for the designated community in each of the following areas:

- Improving health status;
- Addressing the health problems of minorities, the poor and other medically underserved populations, and
- Containing the growth of healthcare costs.

Required characteristics:

CB.2.1 The hospital sponsors projects that are designed to improve the community's health status.
CB.2.1.1 Measurable objectives are specified for these projects to be achieved within a specified time frame.
CB.2.1.2 One project involves an effort to increase awareness and understanding of health status indicators, and the activities that are expected to favorably affect these indicators.
CB.2.1.3 Other projects to accomplish health status objectives may include:
CB.2.1.3.1 Sponsoring disease prevention and/or health education programs.
CB.2.1.3.2 Sponsoring healthcare programs for individuals with special health problems.
CB.2.1.3.3 Sponsoring efforts to improve the community's health through economic and community development.
CB.2.1.3.4 Developing quality assessment programs for community healthcare that currently lack these programs and, if feasible, assisting in their implementation.
CB.2.1.3.5 Implementing other projects to improve community health status.
CB.2.2 The hospital participates in projects to address the health problems of minorities, the poor and other medically underserved populations.
CB.2.2.1 Measurable objectives are specified for these projects to be achieved within a specified time frame.

APPENDIX 2-1. *(Continued)*

CB.2.2.2 One project involves an effort to increase awareness of the special health problems of minorities, the poor and medically underserved populations, and the activities that might address these problems.

CB.2.2.3 Other projects to accomplish these objectives may include:

CB2.2.3.1 Improving accessibility and continuity of care for minorities, the poor and medically underserved populations.

CB.2.2.3.2 Working to reduce the disparities in health status which exist among racial and ethnic minorities.

CB.2.2.3.3 Sponsoring efforts to increase the number of minorities, the poor and medically underserved populations who enter health professions and who work in medically underserved communities.

CB.2.2.3.4 Participating in other activities that address the health problems of minorities, the poor and medically underserved populations.

CB.2.3 The hospital participates in projects that are designed to contain the growth of the community's healthcare costs.

CB.2.3.1 Measurable objectives are specified for these projects to be achieved within a specified time frame.

CB.2.3.2 One project involves an effort to increase awareness of the magnitude and the rate of growth of the community's health-care costs, and the activities that might contain the growth of these costs.

CB.2.3.3 Other projects to accomplish these objectives may include:

CB.2.3.3.1 Improving the efficiency of specified healthcare services.

CB.2.3.3.2 Improving case management and continuity of care for individuals with special healthcare problems.

CB.2.3.3.3 Sponsoring health promotion, disease prevention or self-care activities that lead to the containment of the growth of healthcare costs.

CB.2.3.3.4 Reducing and/or avoiding redundancy of specific healthcare services.

CB.2.3.3.5 Carrying out other activities to contain the growth of healthcare costs.

Standard CB.3 The hospital's program includes activities designed to stimulate other organizations and individuals to join in carrying out a broad health agenda in the designated community.

Required characteristics:

CB.3.1 The hospital cultivates and maintains effective relationships with other healthcare and community organizations to increase

APPENDIX 2-1. *(Continued)*

common awareness and sensitivity to the designated community's healthcare problems.

CB.3.2 The hospital works with others to identify specific community healthcare problems and approaches to their solutions.

CB.3.3 The hospital works with others to assist in the implementation of activities that further a broad community health agenda.

CB.3.4 The hospital encourages the involvement of leaders from the following community groups in fulfilling Required Characteristics CB.3.1 through CB.3.3:

CB.3.4.1 Minorities, the poor and medically underserved populations;

CB.3.4.2 Other hospitals and healthcare organizations;

CB.3.4.3 Other community organizations;

CB.3.4.4 The local public health department and other governmental agencies;

CB3.4.5 Educational institutions;

CB.3.4.6 Physicians, nurses and other health professionals; and

CB.3.4.7 Other individuals as deemed appropriate.

Standard CB.4 The hospital fosters an internal environment that encourages hospitalwide involvement in the program.

Required characteristics:

CB.4.1 The medical staff is appropriately integrated into the activities of the program.

CB.4.1.1 The medical staff organization has a mechanism to encourage medical staff participation in program activities.

CB.4.1.2 Individual members of the medical staff are provided specific opportunities to participate in the activities of the program.

CB.4.2 Hospital employees are appropriately integrated into the activities of the program.

CB.4.2.1 There is a special effort to include those employees who reside in the designated community.

CB.4.2.2 Individual employees are provided specific opportunities to participate in the activities of the program.

CB.4.3 There is a mechanism to foster cooperation among all departments in the hospital that should participate in the program.

CB.4.4 The hospital's volunteer activities are appropriately integrated into the program.

Source: *The Hospital Community Benefits Standards Program* (New York: New York University, 1989). Used with permission.

3

The Six-Step Process for Creating and Building Healthy Communities

Play for more than you can afford to lose, and you will learn the game.

—*Winston Churchill*

M any trustees believe that health care reform must begin on the local level, in the communities that their organizations serve. Trustees are, in fact, in the best position to lead their organizations toward a new vision of health as the creation of healthy communities. Their support and leadership are critical to the success of health care reform initiatives. To become the visionary leaders that health care needs, trustees must re-examine long-held beliefs and values, adopt 21st-century principles of governance, embrace the concept of a healthy community, and develop a systematic approach, or plan, for change.

This chapter describes such a plan. Based on the collective knowledge of boards that have successfully led their organizations through change, the plan consists of a systematic six-step process. Like most contemporary improvement models, the process begins with techniques for creating awareness of the need to change and ends with techniques for measuring and sustaining gains.

OVERVIEW OF THE SIX-STEP PROCESS

"Board members must open their minds to change and do whatever it takes to preserve and enhance the delivery of quality care in their communities. It is truly an exciting and difficult time to be a board member. Working as a team is essential."

The six-step process for creating and building healthy communities describes what boards must do to plan, implement, and evaluate the effectiveness of community health initiatives. (See figure 3-1.) This process is applicable to all types of initiatives, from modest, start-up efforts to comprehensive programs. As the figure shows, the process is continuous; implicit in the model is the belief that experience leads to improvement and that success breeds success. In short, initiatives that improve the health of the community tend to heighten awareness of health issues, this awareness paving the way to further, and often even more effective, initiatives.

The first step of the process—*create awareness of community health issues*—focuses on the need to become familiar with the health status of the community. This step can be accomplished through informal methods, such as community visits, and more formal means, such as community health assessments and benchmark comparisons. Once the board becomes aware of community health issues, then it can knowledgeably engage in step 2—*engage others in dialogue*. This step

FIGURE 3-1. The Six-Step Process

Step 1. *Create awareness of community health issues*

- Conduct a health status assessment
- Identify Benchmark Indicators

Step 2. *Engage others in dialogue*

- Create the environment to engage in dialogue
- Exchange information with potential partners

Step 3. *Collaborate with others*

- Form a core group to actively discuss and engage in problem solving
- Adopt a framework for creating healthy communities

Step 4. *Redesign the system*

- Brainstorm solutions and assign responsibilities
- Form an action plan and implement the action initiative

Step 5. *Evaluate the outcome*

- Evaluate the process
- Measure achievement toward the goal

Step 6. *Sustain the gains*

- Identify the key success factors
- Continually improve upon the gains

involves reaching out to other organizations to talk about the community's unmet health needs. Steps 3 and 4—*collaborate with others and redesign the system*—are the "meat" of the process. During these steps, collaborators exchange information about community health issues and resources, brainstorm solutions to health problems, and formulate and implement a plan of action. Step 5—*evaluate the outcome*—entails reviewing the effectiveness of the planning and implementation process and measuring achievement of goals. During the last step—*sustain the gains*—collaborators identify key success factors to ensure that results already achieved are continuously improved upon.

The remainder of this chapter describes each of the six steps in detail. To facilitate implementation of the process, the chapter explains methods that boards and their organizations can use to complete each step successfully.

STEP 1: CREATE AWARENESS OF COMMUNITY HEALTH ISSUES

"Board members must recognize the difficult but necessary prioritization of community first, organization second."

The first and most important step in the process of creating and building healthy communities is for boards to become aware of the health issues that their communities face. For many governance teams, a community health status assessment is a solid way to create governance and community awareness of health needs. The governance team should authorize management to perform a health status assessment tailored to the organization's service area. To pinpoint which health issues are the most significant, the team might also have management make statistical benchmark comparisons of the health of the service area and other, comparable communities.

The Community Health Status Assessment

According to VHA Inc., a community health assessment is a "dynamic process undertaken to identify the health problems and goals of the community, enable the community-wide establishment of health priorities, and facilitate collaborative action planning directed at improving community health status and quality of life. Involving multiple sectors of the community, the assessment draws upon both quantitative and qualitative population-based health status and health-services utilization data. With strong emphasis on community ownership of the process, a community health assessment supports developing community competence in the identification and response to community health problems and goals."[1]

Board members might start by visiting local neighborhoods to assess the community's health. The board chair of an organization located in an urban community suggested to me that trustees should "tour the neighborhood, get out of the bus, and talk to the people." Other, more structured methods of assessing the community's health are community forums and community profiles.

The Healthy Community Forum The healthy community forum is an assessment technique in which community leaders get together to brainstorm and prioritize community health issues that need to be addressed. (The healthy community forum is similar to the community future search, described in chapter 1.) Depending on the size and composition of the organization's service area, participants might include representatives of key health care organizations; governmental, religious, and charitable organizations; and the local school system and chamber of commerce. For many governance teams, the healthy community forum is an important action step. Because this type of assessment is done in collaboration with other stakeholders, it paves the way to broad-based community involvement and follow-up.

For example, Fairview Hospital and Healthcare Services in Minneapolis, Minnesota, completed such an assessment and found that family violence, especially violence toward children, was affecting the health of the community. Based on this information, Fairview approached the Minnesota Department of Health to collaborate on a prevention initiative with a mission to "ensure a safe and secure family and community environment for children through community-wide efforts aimed at preventing violence." Efforts to eliminate violence in the community are ongoing.

The Community Profile Another useful tool is the community profile. Where the aforementioned healthy community forum can be a useful method for gathering feedback about community health issues, the community profile, in contrast, provides stakeholders with a "snapshot" of the community's position on three levels. First, the profile describes the community's demographics. Second, it maps the capacity of the community in terms of assets and liabilities that can be brought to bear on a particular health issue. (The "capacity" of a community can be thought of as the community's ability to work through and resolve its health issues.) Third, it maps the capability and the relationships of the local associations and institutions that can be mobilized for a particular health issue.

Benchmark Indicators

Benchmark indicators are another useful way to gather information about the status of the community's health. Through the use of standardized measures, benchmarking can help pinpoint specific areas of concern. The following benchmark indicators are especially helpful in heightening awareness of unmet community health needs:

- infant mortality rate per 1,000
- pregnancy rate per 1,000 girls 10–17 years old
- number of aggravated assaults per 100,000 people as reported to the police or service providers
- number of rapes per 100,000 women as reported to the police or service providers
- number of violence-related deaths due to homicides per 100,000 under 30 years of age
- number of children ages 0–6 years old with elevated blood lead levels
- percentage of pregnant women completing recommended prenatal care
- percentage of low-birth-weight babies (< 2,500 grams)
- percentage of children ages 0–6 who have completed all recommended basic immunization series
- primary care providers per 100,000 people in the state
- number of deaths caused by unintentional injuries per 100,000 population
- total health care expenses per capita
- health care expenses as a percent of the gross state product

The chair of one board requested the adoption of a series of benchmark indicators to determine how the health status of the organization's community compared to other communities and to determine the high-risk, high-profile, high-leverage areas the organization could focus on to make a difference. When the statistics were reviewed at the next meeting, the board discovered that the community had one of the highest infant mortality rates in the country. The board also discovered that the community had higher percentages of low-birth-weight babies and babies born to teens, which resulted in greater utilization of the neonatal intensive care unit. One board member commented, "Maybe if we spend more on prenatal care and sex education, we could avoid the lengthy and costly stays in the neonatal intensive care unit." As a result, the board's focus turned to community intervention initiatives aimed at decreasing the rate of teen pregnancy. The board conducted a health status assessment, identified a gap, investigated best practices from other communities, and ultimately decreased teen pregnancy in the community. In this case, board awareness of a community health problem led to both reduced costs and a healthier community.

A List of Ideas for Your Next Board Meeting

Community health assessments and benchmarking are just two of many tools available to heighten awareness of community health issues. Figure 3-2 cites other resources, from literature searches to healthy community indexes (which identify a community's problem-solving capactiy and serve as self-evaluations of a community's strengths and weaknesses). To initiate discussion about health issues in your own community, bring the following list of ideas to your next board meeting:

- Ask management if a health status assessment has ever been conducted in the communities you serve.
- Contact local and state health departments to see if they have information about the health status of the organization's service area.
- Do a community health inventory. Invite other nonprofit organizations and the business community to take an inventory of what others are doing to improve the health of the community. Or ask management to determine the level of interest in your own community for this type of assessment.
- Conduct a literature search to see what other communities across the country have done to create greater awareness of health issues.
- Ask for a comparison of the cost of selective prevention initiatives compared to the cost of acute medical interventions.
- Actively discuss your community's health issues.

STEP 2: ENGAGE OTHERS IN DIALOGUE

> "We must listen to what the public wants, discuss how it could happen in our facilities, and continually work to fulfill the needs of our communities."

No single health care organization or sector of the community can successfully identify and work through its health issues in isolation. The involvement of multiple stakeholders is crucial to long-term success. The

FIGURE 3-2. Ways to Create Awareness

• vital records	• benchmark indicators
• community surveys	• health statistics
• literature search	• demographic profile
• community health inventory	• prevention initiatives
• health status assessment	• healthy community index
• morbidity and mortality indices	• census information

second step in the process of building healthier communities is, then, to engage others in a dialogue about how to move the process forward.

As the model in figure 3-3 shows, there is a world of difference between true dialogue and the kind of discussion in which leaders often engage. Edgar H. Schein, the creator of the model, points out that "the essential concept underlying dialogue [is] the discovery of one's own internal choice process regarding when to speak and what to say."[2] The model is a gentle reminder about the choices leaders have when they enter into conversation with others. Leaders can waste time in debate, or they can leave egos and vested interests behind, suspend old assumptions and agendas, and work together for the common good. The choice is clear: Those who engage in dialogues about com-

FIGURE 3-3. Ways of Talking Together

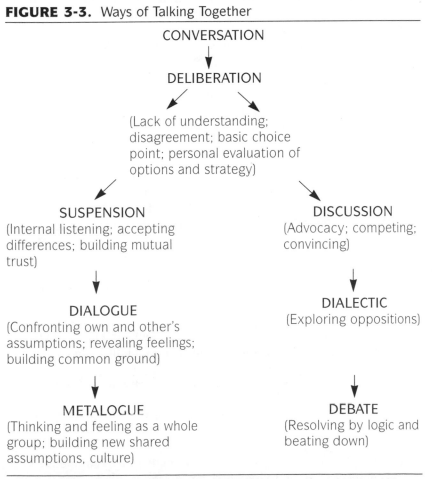

munity health should view themselves as partners in problem solving. Their sole purpose should be to improve the heath care delivery system and the health status of the community.

Three Factors That Facilitate Dialogue

Three factors that contribute to true dialogue and subsequent action are governance team leadership, agreement among participants on a common goal, and the development of trust. The three factors are described below.

Governance Team Leadership   True leaders are willing to talk to potential partners, even if those partners have traditionally been competitors. Some board members who have participated in healthy community initiatives suggest that the governance teams of competing organizations meet informally to find and reach common ground. One board member who chaired a community service committee said to me, "We talked to several competing health care organizations—they had been in the community for almost one hundred years—and we found we both had the same community interests in mind. Our assessments showed the same findings, so we decided to work together to solve the issue of prenatal care and access to primary care. It's working."

Agreement on a Common Goal   The second factor that facilitates dialogue is agreement on a common goal or goals. When different parties sit at the table, it is easier for them to engage in true dialogue if they share a common purpose. Consider the example of two board chairs who believed that their communities would be better off if their health care organizations would only work together, stop the duplication of technology and services, and work toward a common purpose of "rationalizing health care in the community and improving the health and quality of life for its citizens." The board chairs agreed on the following course of action:

- monthly breakfast meetings of the board chairs and their CEOs
- determination of organizational similarities and differences
- focus on similarities and common ground
- dialogues about low-risk, high-potential activities of community benefit
- quarterly reports to respective boards on the progress of the dialogues

After two years of regular meetings between these two competitors, the board chairs shared the following observations:

Our first series of breakfasts dealt with a lot of old history. Each organization jockeyed for position. At about the second quarter mark, we better understood each other's organizations but we also got to know each other personally. We started by agreeing to use the Hospital Community Benefits Program [see chapter 2] as our framework to engage in a dialogue. We eventually combined our ethics committees, held joint educational sessions between our boards and management, and eventually committed to expand our partnership to work on issues that were unique to our community. We talked to service organizations, the United Way, the chamber of commerce, the business community, and others to begin to understand our community health issues. We eventually worked collectively to resolve issues such as access to care, teen pregnancy, and injury prevention among our younger population. From humble beginnings, major transformation that benefited the community occurred.

Development of Trust The third factor that facilitates dialogue is trust, the glue that holds relationships together. Trust is developed by "walking the talk," that is, behaving in a manner consistent with expressed beliefs.

The development of trust can take time, particularly when competitors come together to form a new relationship. As the chair describes the breakfast meetings above, initially competitiveness tarnished the meetings, until a few months into the relationship when the chairs developed a personal relationship. At this point, they knew each other well enough to set aside hidden agendas and develop a trusting relationship.

When different stakeholders develop trust in each other, true transformation often takes place. Consider the example of Mercy Health Services in Farmington, Michigan, which performed a health status assessment in 1989. The assessment used face-to-face surveys and focus groups that included residents and service providers from the community. The major issues identified in the study were jobs and unemployment, health, education, housing, and crime. Mercy Hospital, along with two hospitals from the east side of Detroit, retained an independent party to conduct a focus group of community leaders regarding the needs of the community and the role Mercy Hospital and others should take in addressing these issues. As a result, a number of sharcholders were identified, each of whom demonstrated a commitment to improving the quality of life in the community. These concerned parties engaged in dialogue, developed trust in each other, and made a difference in improving the health of the population on the east side of Detroit.[3]

A List of Ideas for Your Next Board Meeting

As you prepare to engage in dialogue with others for the purpose of building a healthier community, you might take any of several actions. Below is a list of ideas to bring to your next board meeting:

- Brainstorm a list of potential partners with whom you might engage in dialogue. The list of stakeholders in figure 3-4 is a good starting point.
- Talk about sponsoring a healthy community future search (described in chapter 1) to kick off the healthy community initiative.
- Create an inventory of the health-related issues in your community and those organizations engaged in their resolution.
- Give each board member a copy of Roger Fisher and William Ury's *Getting to Yes*, which is about the negotiating process.[4]
- Identify your competitors and ask where there may be areas of concern or mutual interest on issues relating to the health of the community.
- Engage the services of a community facilitator to bring about successful dialogue.

Governance teams should remember that all communities are made up of interdependent segments. What happens in each influences the health of the whole. Dialogue helps boards better understand their connection to the community. For every board, there is a whole community just waiting to be explored.

STEP 3: COLLABORATE WITH OTHERS

"Twenty-first-century governance must be a team effort, from top to bottom."

Once boards have become familiar with community health issues and engaged in meaningful dialogue with others, they are ready for collabora-

FIGURE 3-4. Potential Partners

• libraries	• cultural organizations
• competitors	• community stakeholders
• city and state government	• chamber of commerce
• public health department	• business and industry
• nonprofit organizations	• churches
• school system	• United Way
• police department	• foundations

tion. As discussed in chapter 2, collaboration involves exchanging information, sharing human and financial resources, and otherwise enhancing the capacity of others to achieve a common vision. In short, this is the step during which boards begin to build bridges to the community.

Key Success Factors

Analysis of collaborations to improve community health show that certain factors are critical to success. One such factor is to include diverse segments of the community; collaboration cannot succeed if essential stakeholders are missing from the table. Once appropriate parties have been brought together, it is important to identify a core group of participants who can develop work processes and plans. Finally, many successful collaborators have found that adoption of a community health framework facilitates planning.

Inclusion of Diverse Community Groups Many communities include diverse demographic groups. If true collaboration is to occur, it is critical that representatives of all segments of the population affected by a health problem be included in the collaboration process. The importance of this factor is illustrated by the success of the Arizona initiative Women to Women. This volunteer outreach program, which grew out of a 1993 meeting between representatives of Tucson Medical Center and a community team, is designed to provide culturally sensitive, easily obtainable health education and support to the women of Pima County. The collaborators who participated in the development of the program reflected the diversity of the community. Represented were teenagers, Hispanics, African Americans, Native Americans, insurers, health professionals, researchers, legislators, teachers, and community volunteers. Women to Women empowered volunteers to be experts in their own community.[5] Collaboration among diverse groups became key to the success of this initiative.

Formation of Core Work Team Once partners have been identified, a core group should be formed to develop work processes and ensure that appropriate organizations and individuals are involved. Often, this core group includes one or two board members. Sharing their unique perspectives, team members engage in problem solving and action planning. For example, a coalition of area hospitals, health agencies, community colleges, businesses, and government agencies formed a core leadership team to launch its planning process. The team systematically prioritized community health problems using three criteria: the magnitude of the problem, the seriousness of the problem, and the feasibility of alleviating the problem. On the basis of these criteria, the core group pinpointed three health problems and designed services and prevention programs to help solve them. One board member from an area hospital stated, "Our core group effectively and efficiently identified our health priorities and actively engaged itself in how to resolve its health problems. We decided to offer services and prevention programs aimed at resolving our community's most critical health concerns."

Adoption of Framework Finally, it often is easier to collaborate successfully if participants adopt a framework for creating healthy communities. The frameworks described in chapter 2 can help collaborators move, in a structured way, closer to community health. One chair suggested that the frameworks help boards to "define the healthy community initiative and commit to a formal process of working with others to improve the health of our community." Many health care organizations that have initiated a course of action to create healthy communities have used one of these frameworks to do so. Other organizations have adopted the Community Care Network vision, described in the preface, to promote health while managing within fixed resources.

A List of Ideas for Your Next Board Meeting

In preparation for collaboration with others, use the following list of ideas to generate discussion at your next board meeting:

- Discuss the staircase of citizen participation depicted in figure 2-3, chapter 2. Where along the staircase would you place your organization and your community?
- Discuss actions to be taken. The list of actions in figure 3-5 might help to focus the discussion.
- Examine the health status assessment and identify one issue and brainstorm the list of potential partners to bring to an issues forum.
- Use The Healthcare Forum Community Builder to engage in a dialogue and assist in the collaborative process. The Community Builder is a strategic simulation designed to engage participants in team-oriented learning by immersing them in developing strategies for improving quality of life.
- Encourage and support collaborative efforts among area health care providers and others that will improve the health of the community.
- Educate the board on collaborative and process improvement techniques to ensure that trustees are trained facilitators.

The process of collaborating often leads boards to develop new skills. Among these skills are the ability to design new organizational forms and processes.

FIGURE 3-5. Collaboration Action Steps

- educate
- share resources
- prioritize health problems
- form a core group
- create partnerships
- create common ground
- set common goals
- clarify expectations
- understand cultural contexts

- work together
- engage in problem solving
- create the environment
- build trust
- adopt a framework
- assign responsibilities
- work with competitors
- set time frames

STEP 4: REDESIGN THE SYSTEM

"Boards must prepare to break from tradition."

Redesigning the system is the most creative part of the healthy community process. Collaborators brainstorm solutions, go on site visits, benchmark with other communities, and eventually form an action plan tailored to the community. The challenge is to design or reinvent a system of care and service that meets the health needs of the population.

Goals of the Redesign

During the redesign, participants engage in a number of activities. (See figure 3-6.) Unmet health needs are clarified, and the core team develops an action plan to close the gaps. Partnerships are created, and new work groups are formed to implement action steps. In summary, the goals of the redesign are as follows:

- Clearly define the health problem and identify its causes.
- Clarify work roles and responsibilities.
- Create a clear action plan.
- Develop a program, service, or product that improves the health status of a large number of people.

Definition of the Problem and Its Causes Through dialogue and collaboration, participants should define a health problem to be solved and the factors causing the problem. In this way, they can ensure that their redesign efforts address the roots of the problem. Identification of causes may take time and effort. One board member told me, "I thought the resolution to the problem we were having relating to an increased number of compromised babies in the neonatal intensive care unit was earlier prenatal intervention." However, after a thorough investigation

FIGURE 3-6. Activities Involved in Redesign

- mobilize resources
- improve health status
- create tangible results
- create an action plan
- affect a large number of people
- create new forms
- develop the economy

- renew the community
- form new partnerships
- resolve broad health issues
- find a common ground
- define the problem
- identify causes of the problem
- brainstorm solutions

of the causes of the problem—poor housing, unemployment, and low self-esteem among young women in the community—the group decided to focus on promoting home ownership, welfare-to-work, and self-esteem programs. Because these programs addressed the real causes of the problem, the number of young mothers delivering low-birth-weight babies was reduced. One obstetrician/gynecologist board member summed up the success of the initiative in two words: "It worked."

Clarification of Work Roles and Responsibilities Because redesign efforts are likely to involve a number of organizations and individuals, it also is critical that participants know who is responsible for what. Clarification of participants' roles and responsibilities can save substantial time and effort. Consider the example of five organizations fiscally supporting a comprehensive healthy community initiative. Collectively, the organizations committed $10 million to the initiative. Because of the amount of the investment, the boards needed to ensure that the money went to the intended initiative and that it leveraged additional investments. Therefore, members of the board of each of the five organizations formed an advisory group to the healthy community initiative. In this case, board members clarified their responsibilities and roles.

Creation of an Action Plan The third goal of a redesign effort is to create a clear action plan. This plan should include a time frame and enough detail to ensure that progress can be measured at quarterly board meetings.

The following example demonstrates the effectiveness of such an action plan. In Detroit, Henry Ford Health System made a commitment to "develop focused strategies that reach beyond our walls to serve those in the community, while at the same time seeking to improve the conditions and behaviors that lead to injury and ill health." To address the challenges of poverty, substance abuse, and violence, Henry Ford Health System developed an action plan, setting measurable goals and the time frame in which the goals should be completed. This action plan clarified the problem, indicated a clear path of action, and eventually created the Center for Integrated Urban Health. The health system defined the role of the center and implemented 13 school-based health programs and an initiative aimed at reducing violence among young people.[6]

Development of the Program or Service Finally, the redesign effort should result in a program, service, or product that meets the needs of the community. A good example of such a program is Healthy Valley 2000, which serves a community in Connecticut. Launched in 1994 after more than a year of planning, Healthy Valley 2000 is designed to meet the needs of Ansonia, Beacon Falls, Derby, Oxford, Seymour, and Shelton, towns with a combined population of 96,000 and an area of 100 square miles. The core group that manages the project is the Stakeholder Committee, which is made up of more than 200 members of the valley community who represent major cultural, social, and regional groups. The purpose of Healthy Valley 2000 is to make the valley a better place in which to live, work, and raise a family by measurably improving the quality of life and health of the community and its residents. Healthy Valley 2000 is also designed to support regional economic development by making the community an attractive place for businesses to locate and for their employees to live. Healthy Valley 2000, the most comprehensive initiative ever undertaken in the community, is intended to create "a blueprint that will guide and position the community in the next century. Healthy Valley 2000 is about mobilizing and empowering the community to solve its own problems and build on existing strengths and resources."[7]

In this case, fundamental changes were made because of broad-based community participation. Systems are often redesigned through this kind of community problem-solving vehicle.

A List of Ideas for Your Next Board Meeting

As you contemplate redesigning systems in your community, bring the following list to generate ideas at your next board meeting:

- What health need was identified in our community health status assessment?
- What are the causes?
- What are the best ways to meet this need?
- What role should our organization play as we begin to improve the health of the population we serve?
- Is there a grand vision we might realize that we previously thought was impossible?

- Is the action plan reasonable and implementable?
- What have other communities done to redesign the system?
- What tangible results will occur as a result of this step in the process?
- What level of financial and human resources is needed? What is our organization willing to commit?

In summary, the redesign step of the healthy community process provides an opportunity to experiment and to learn from other communities facing similar issues. It also is the step during which tangible results are seen.

STEP 5: EVALUATE THE OUTCOME

"Institutions can launch initiative after initiative, but if they don't assess progress and outcomes, their innovations will fall flat."

After a community health initiative has been launched, it is important to evaluate the process used to develop and implement the initiative as well as the specific outcomes of the initiative itself. Unfortunately, this step is often overlooked. One veteran of community program development said to me, "We spend an inordinate amount of time planning and launching new healthy community initiatives, but we never spend time post-launch evaluating the outcome. We never know what's worked and what hasn't worked." To understand what works in order to repeat it, it is essential to evaluate the process and measure achievement toward the goal.

A Checklist for Evaluating the Process and Outcomes

The following checklist consists of questions that the core team can use to evaluate the planning and implementation process. A team member should be assigned the responsibility for coordinating the evaluation and ensuring that feedback from all particpants is solicited. A final evaluation report should then be presented to the stakeholders and should be available in writing to the core team members. Responses to these questions should be recorded and saved so that they can be used to direct future efforts.

- Were appropriate stakeholders included in the process?
- Was leadership of the process truly shared?
- What were the strengths and weaknesses of the process?

- Were assignments and responsibilities clear?
- Did core team members work together productively?
- What would we do differently?
- What would we do the same?
- Were the community's priorities clear?

In addition to evaluating the process, it is important to ask whether the goal or goals of the initiative were achieved. The overriding question to ask is, Did the program, service, or product measurably improve the health status of the community? When outcomes are measured, it is also important to ask how effectively the following resources were mobilized:

- information
- fiscal support
- community residents and volunteers
- members of the business community
- local and state government agencies
- other stakeholders

A List of Questions for Your Next Board Meeting

By evaluating outcomes of community initiatives, participants demonstrate a willingness to learn together as a community. There is intrinsic value in this learning process.

Bring the following list of questions to the next board meeting devoted to evaluation of an initiative:

- What worked?
- What didn't work?
- What were the weaknesses of the process?
- What results were achieved?
- How did the health status of the community improve?
- What group process was used?
- Were resources effectively mobilized?
- Were new partnerships effective?
- What were the strengths of the process?
- Did we achieve our goal?

STEP 6: SUSTAIN THE GAINS

"Now that we've fully grasped the health issues facing our community and have begun taking active steps toward creating a community-wide wellness plan, one of our biggest challenges is avoiding complacency. Although we've jumped many hurdles, the race is far from over."

Once a healthy community process or initiative is up and running, it is important to sustain and continually improve upon the gains. To monitor progress, the governance team should ask management to provide, on a quarterly basis, reports that outline progress towards specified goals, key success factors, and a year-to-date assessment. Table 3-1 illustrates a simple and useful reporting system. The key success factors outlined in the model are based on statistical indicators related to the community health problems to be addressed. In addition, most of the health care organizations researched for this book achieved sustainable actions and gains primarily though the use of three methods:

1. periodically assessing, monitoring, and evaluating the board's performance in the area of creating healthy communities
2. charging a governance committee with responsibility for community service
3. developing financial strategies and partnerships

TABLE 3-1. Model of a Reporting System

Goal	Key Success Factors	Year-to-Date Assessment
Create a healthy population	*Statistical factors* • primary care providers per 100,000 population • infant mortality rate • percentage of pregnant women completing prenatal care	
	Project status • primary care health center • school-based clinics	
	Leadership • achieve goals of the governance community service committee • healthy community forum and follow-up	

Periodic Assessment, Monitoring, and Evaluation

In many organizations, the governance team is assigned the responsibility of monitoring and evaluating the board's performance in the area of creating healthy communities. Often, self-assessment tools were used as part of the board evaluation. The self-assessment survey (appendix 3-1 at the end of this chapter) can be used as a stand-alone tool or as part of a larger board self-evaluation process. The survey items address the board's key roles and responsibilities in community health oversight.

To use the survey for assessment purposes, each trustee should independently and anonymously rate the board's performance on each of the items. All responses should then be compiled and analyzed. Particular attention should be paid to items for which there is significant variance in ratings (some trustees rating performance very high while others rate it very low) and to items that receive predominantly negative responses. The overall results of the survey should then be discussed with the board as a whole. Finally, on the basis of the discussion, the board should create an action plan to increase the effectiveness of its oversight and improvement of the health of the communities served.[8]

Formation of a Governance Community Service Committee

A second method of sustaining gains is to form a community service committee. The committee, which typically includes at-large community representatives, can provide an important link to the organization's service area. One board chair told me, "Our community service committee allowed us to monitor the pulse of the community and proved to be the prime way of creating healthy populations." In many instances, this committee not only provides the principal link to the community but also educates the board on the health status of the populations served by the organization. More specifically, the committee might be charged with fulfilling the following responsibilities:

- creating a strategy for realizing the organization's healthy community vision
- monitoring institutional priorities relative to the strategy
- providing financial oversight of investments for healthy community initiatives
- educating the board on the health status of the community and opportunities to improve health status
- identifying community contacts and opportunities for community involvement that are linked to the vision and mission

- assisting in developing in-kind partnerships for programs and services that benefit the community

Development of Financial Strategies and Partnerships

A third method of achieving sustainable gains is to develop financial strategies and long-term partnerships. All the health care organizations researched for this book made a financial commitment to creating healthier communities. Those that sustained community health initiatives over the long term often did so through financial strategies. Many more sustained gains through a partnership strategy.

Memorial Hospital and Health System To help finance outreach programs, Memorial Hospital and Health System, Inc., in South Bend, Indiana, uses a tithing approach called "the 10 Percent Solution." With this approach, the hospital has agreed to reserve 10 percent of its previous year's surplus of funds. This amount is then applied to programs that meet the following nine criteria:

- fulfillment of the mission of the hospital
- service of an identified, unmet need in the community
- collaboration with other community providers or organizations
- reasonable cost
- "new" programs or "above and beyond" efforts of existing programs
- incorporation of quality improvement principles with defined measurable outcomes
- preventive and educational focus
- service to the system's constituency
- proposal and management by Memorial

Programs usually include nonacute care services that improve the community's health status and educate or provide social services to the elderly, children, medically indigent, and other targeted groups. Examples of such programs are health screenings, community health or disease-specific educational activities, immunization services, temporary housing, transportation, basic science and research, volunteer services, and medical education.

Chicago's Mount Sinai Medical Center Since 1983, Mount Sinai Medical Center in Chicago has supported neighborhood redevelopment efforts through partnerships with others. With Ryerson Steel Company, the medical center pledged $600,000 in operating funds and raised $100,000 from local businesses every year for seven years to open a housing and renovation agency, the Neighborhood Housing Services. Mount Sinai also joined with Neighborhood Housing Services, the Metropolitan Housing Development Corporation, and a private home builder in the New Homes for Chicago project, which obtained a $400,000 subsidy from the city to build 20 affordable single-family houses. The project also sought out lending institutions that would provide low-interest loans to purchase the homes for families with annual incomes of less than $30,000.

In further neighborhood redevelopment initiatives, Mount Sinai convinced the city of Chicago to repave local streets and provide new sidewalks and curbs for 70 of the approximately 100 blocks of the surrounding neighborhood. In conjunction with city officials, Mount Sinai also encouraged the state government to fund the modernization of the thoroughfare that links Mount Sinai with the University of Illinois at Chicago health complex.[9]

Hartford Childhood Immunization Program In Hartford, Connecticut, the Hartford Childhood Immunization Program was funded in 1992 by a $1 million grant from the Aetna Foundation. The Program mandates a statewide registry of children born in Connecticut in order to establish a tracking system for immunization. The Aetna Foundation, M.D. Health Plan, and Connecticut Children's Medical Center purchased a mobile health screening and immunization van that provides immunizations to children who may not otherwise be immunized.

A List of Ideas for Your Next Board Meeting

As the initiatives in the case examples show, gains are sustained when boards generate both financial and human resource support from key segments of the community. It is also important to note that many of the successful initiatives focused on creating a stronger economy or a more healthful environment. Boards must understand that the state of the local economy and neighborhood has a direct impact on the state of the community's health. (See figure 3-7.) Below is a list of ideas and questions to bring to your next board meeting as you think about ways to sustain community gains:

- What is our board's level of commitment, both human and fiscal, to the healthy community initiative?
- What is the most effective way to share the leadership for the healthy community initiative?
- How do we sustain the process?

FIGURE 3-7. Two Views of Health

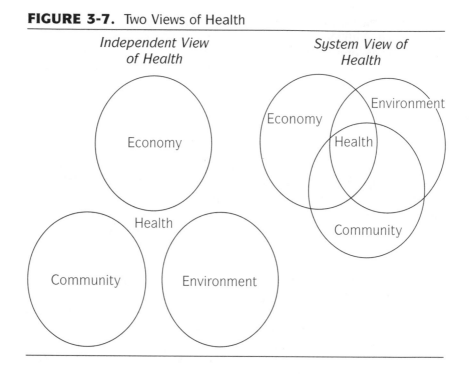

- How do we continually improve what we have today?
- What is our next community initiative?

The best and most effective way of sustaining the gains is to invest in the community's future and to continuously build upon the process and outcomes of the healthy community initiatives.

CONCLUSION

If boards really believe that "health happens out there," as one board chair told me, then they must connect with the players out there. One obstacle stands in their way: a credibility problem. Americans have a low level of confidence in their health care organizations. According to *Second Opinions*, a publication of the Public Agenda Foundation, only 41 percent of Americans have "a great deal" or "quite a lot" of confidence in their hospitals and clinics.[10] Local business leaders, local government, state and federal government, national business leaders, and political parties all ranked behind hospitals and clinics.

What does this crisis in confidence mean to trustees? It means that one of their most important constituents may not be open to forming the close partnership necessary to improve community health. The only way to overcome this credibility problem is to develop new relationships and broad-based community forums. The six-step process for creating and building healthy communities provides a model for boards to reach out to their communities.

References

1. Christina Bethell, *Community Health Assessment: A Process for Positive Change* (Irving, Tex.: VHA, Inc., 1993), p. 25.

2. Edgar H. Schein, "On Dialogue, Culture, and Organizational Learning," *Organizational Dynamics* 22, no. 2 (1993): 45.

3. Brenita Crawford (President and CEO), "Developing a Community Benefit Plan for an Urban Community Health Care System" (Mercy Hospital, Farmington, Mich., 1994), p. 2.

4. R. Fisher and W. Ury, *Getting to Yes: Negotiating Agreement without Giving In* (Boston: Houghton Mifflin, 1983).

5. Tucson Medical Center, "Women to Women Community Prenatal Outreach" (Tucson, Ariz., 1994), p. 2.

6. Henry Ford Health System, *Reaching Out to the Community* (Detroit, Mich.: Henry Ford Health System, 1997), p. 2.

7. *Healthy Valley 2000 Annual Report, 1994–1995* (Ansonia, Conn.: Healthy Valley 2000, 1995), p. 7.

8. James E. Orlikoff and Mary K. Totten, "Trustee Workbook #2: Assessing and Improving Your Community's Health," *Trustee* 48, no. 5 (1995).

9. Karen Sandrick, "If You Want to Play, You've Got to Pay," *Hospitals and Health Networks* (July 1995): 26.

10. John Immerwaher and Jean Johnson, *Second Opinions: Americans' Changing Views on Healthcare Reform* (New York: The Public Agenda Foundation, 1994).

APPENDIX 3-1. A Self-Assessment Questionnaire

1. The mission of our organization reflects a strong commitment to the community and to the assessment and improvement of the health of the community.
   ☐ Yes   ☐ No

2. Our community is clearly defined.
   ☐ Yes   ☐ No

3. The board is an effective link between the hospital and the community.
   ☐ strongly agree   ☐ agree
   ☐ disagree   ☐ strongly disagree

4. Community organizations/leaders are regularly consulted about the value of the organization's services.
   ☐ strongly agree   ☐ agree
   ☐ disagree   ☐ strongly disagree

5. Board members are active spokespeople in the community about health care issues.
   ☐ strongly agree   ☐ agree
   ☐ disagree   ☐ strongly disagree

6. We regularly assess and can readily demonstrate that our organization provides a high level of benefit to our community.
   ☐ strongly agree   ☐ agree
   ☐ disagree   ☐ strongly disagree

7. The community benefit is regularly measured and quantified, and exceeds in dollar value the amount of savings our organization annually realizes from our tax exemption.
   ☐ strongly agree   ☐ agree
   ☐ disagree   ☐ strongly disagree

8. There is a strong, trusting relationship between our organization and at least three community organizations in partnering to assess and improve the health of our communities.
   ☐ strongly agree   ☐ agree
   ☐ disagree   ☐ strongly disagree

9. We have a detailed plan with our partners to assess and improve the health of our community.
   ☐ strongly agree   ☐ agree
   ☐ disagree   ☐ strongly disagree

10. Our new board member orientation process includes a session on community health and the board's responsibility for it.
   ☐ strongly agree   ☐ agree
   ☐ disagree   ☐ strongly disagree

Source: James E. Orlikoff and Mary K. Totten, "Trustee Workbook #2: Assessing and Improving Your Community's Health," *Trustee* 48, no. 5 (May 1995). Reprinted with permission.

4

The Five Core Competencies of Highly Effective Boards

I know of no safe repository of the ultimate powers of the society but the people themselves; and if we think them not enlightened enough to exercise control with a wholesome discretion, the remedy is not to take it from them, but to inform their discretion by education.

—*Thomas Jefferson*

There is a strong correlation between an organization's ability to create and build healthy communities and the effectiveness of its governance. The effective governance system around which this book is built has outlined a path that boards can follow to strengthen both the organizations they lead and the communities they serve. The first building block of the system—the five principles of contemporary governance (see chapter 1)—familiarized boards with cutting-edge governance theory. The second building block—the six-step process for creating and building healthy communities (see chapter 3)—translated theory into practice. This chapter presents the final building block of the effective governance system—five core competencies of highly effective boards.

My research has shown that a significant gap exists between current and 21st-century governance practices. (See appendix A at the end of this book.) The governance survey I conducted pointed to five core competencies that separate the 20th-century board from the 21st-century board:

- *community stewardship:* creating healthy communities, focusing on the health status of the population, and serving the public
- *visionary leadership:* leaving the past behind, picturing what a better future might look like, and articulating that picture in words

67

- *systems thinking:* seeing the interrelationship between what boards and their organizations do and the health of the communities they serve
- *high-leverage actions:* becoming change masters, practicing effective strategic planning, and communicating effectively
- *basic business skills:* striving for cost-effectiveness, quality improvement, and increased productivity

By building these competencies, boards can bridge the gap between traditional governance and 21st-century leadership.

COMMUNITY STEWARDSHIP

"The board should be a positive force and a leader in the community. Its members should act as an arm of the organization that is accessible to the community and receptive to feedback."

As chapter 1 pointed out, governance teams must move from trusteeship of the organization to stewardship of the community. There is a world of difference between these two approaches to governance. In the words of Peter Block, "Stewardship holds the possibility of shifting expectations of people in power. Part of the meaning of stewardship is to hold in trust the well being of some larger entity—our organizations, our community, the earth itself. To hold something of value in trust calls for placing service ahead of control, to no longer expect leaders to be in charge and out in front. There is pride in leadership, it evokes images of direction. There is humility in stewardship, it evokes images of service. Service is central to the idea of stewardship."[1]

To become stewards of community health, boards must understand that the answers to the health issues facing our communities can be found within the communities themselves. Stewardship thus requires a fundamental shift in both control and power. When boards embrace stewardship, service and outcome become more important to them than ownership, and shared power becomes more important than control of the process. Community stewardship entails three important actions: creating healthy communities, focusing on the health status of the population, and serving the public.

The Creation of Healthy Communities

Traditionally, health care organizations have been guided by a narrow definition of health. By adopting a broader definition of health, which encompasses quality-of-life issues, governance teams will find new and exciting opportunities for improving the health status of the communities they serve.

A Broader Definition of Health According to *Second Opinion*, a study issued by The Public Agenda Foundation, "There is a difference between healthcare and health itself. Many of the cases of ill health are social and cultural (smoking and substance abuse, violent crime) and do not respond directly to changes in healthcare policy."[2] To get the public's perspective on this issue, The Public Agenda asked a representative sampling of Americans to rate the relative importance of three determinants of health: personal responsibility (taking care of oneself), biology (age, genes, and other physical characteristics), and access to good medical care. Most respondents (57 percent) said that an individual's own actions were the most important factor in determining health. Only 21 percent thought that biological factors beyond one's control were the most important factor, while access to good medical care was a distant third, with only 14 percent of respondents indicating that this was the most important factor.

Similar results were found when respondents rated eight factors that keep people healthy. "Taking care of one's self" was at the top of the list, with 84 percent saying that this factor "helps a lot," followed by controlling pollution (67 percent), reducing violence (63 percent), and having a supportive, nonstressful job and family life (60 percent). Respondents indicated that access to medical care (having health insurance or getting frequent diagnostic tests) was less important in contributing to overall health. In fact, living near first-rate hospitals was at the bottom of respondents' lists, with only 30 percent saying that this "helps a lot" in keeping people healthy.[3] The clear message from the American public is that health can only be improved by moving beyond our traditional medical boundaries.

An Emerging Model of Health Care To move beyond traditional boundaries, governance teams must be willing to take a proactive stance toward health. That means keeping apace with the enormous changes that have been occurring in health care. Charles E. Exley, a former chairman and CEO of National Cash Register, once observed, "When you are in the business of making milk bottles and someone discovers milk cartons, you've got a real problem!"[4] Many of our health care organizations are still making milk bottles. To keep apace of change, governance teams must redefine health care as a system of optimizing community health, and organizations must shift their focus from procedure and complication management to the care of covered lives or the health of geographic populations. When our governance teams redefine health care in its broadest sense, then a new model of care delivery will emerge. (See figure 4-1.)

The new model of care includes assessing the health status of the population, implementing a case management system of delivering care from pre- to posthospital care, offering a range of health promotion initiatives, and managing the course of disease and health over the lifetime of the populations served. Naturally, health care organizations will continue to admit patients for care, but in the future, inpatients will represent a smaller component of the care system.

Focus on the Health Status of the Population

To become stewards of the community, boards also must become familiar with health indicators, such as the leading causes of death and the lifestyle factors that contribute to them. Evidence compiled by the Centers for Disease Control and the U.S. Department of Health and Human Services shows that lifestyle factors lead to half of the 10 leading medical causes of death. (See table 4-1.) It is therefore reasonable to assume that providing education to the community and combating such health problems as tobacco use will lead to better community health.

The health status of every community can be measured; thus, health status indicators should be a part of every governance team's new toolbox. State and local public health departments provide a rich source of information about the health status of the population. The following sections note some useful tools and resources for governance teams.

Social Indicators III   This publication, created by the U.S. Department of Commerce, presents "an extensive set of social indicators in the areas of population and family; health and nutrition; housing and environment; transportation; public safety; education and training; work; Social Security and welfare; income and productivity; social participation; culture, leisure and use of time."[5]

FIGURE 4-1. Improving the Health of the Population

Covered lives/geographic population

Health status assessment system

Case management system

Health promotion

Disease/health management

Complication management

TABLE 4-1. Causes of Death Linked to Lifestyle Factors

The 10 leading medical causes of death . . .	
Heart disease	720,000
Cancer	505,000
Cerebrovascular disease	144,000
Accidents	92,000
Chronic pulmonary disease	87,000
Pneumonia and influenza	80,000
Diabetes	48,000
Suicide	31,000
Liver disease, cirrhosis	26,000
AIDS	25,000
Total	2,148,000
. . . and lifestyle factors leading to half of them	
Tobacco	400,000
Diet; sedentary lifestyle	300,000
Alcohol	100,000
Infections	90,000
Toxic agents	60,000
Firearms	35,000
Sexual behavior	30,000
Motor vehicles	25,000
Illicit drug use	20,000
Total	1,060,000

Source: Department of Health and Human Services, Centers for Disease Control, National Center for Health Statistics, Hyattsville, Md., 1996.

The Rand-McNally Guide to the Best Places to Live in America This popular and useful book ranks 329 metropolitan areas in the categories of climate and terrain, housing, health care and environment, crime, transportation, education, the arts, recreation, and economics.[6]

The Prevention Index This publication is an assessment of personal preventive behavior. The Prevention Research Center has also developed an index to assess the extent to which communities take "affirmative action steps for preventing disease and promoting health by creating a community environment."[7]

Healthy People 2000 Healthy People 2000 was established by the U.S. Public Health Service, which developed a comprehensive set of determinants to enable communities to measure health status. It uses health status indicators that enable communities to measure health status outcomes and make national comparisons over time. According to the U.S. Public Health Service, "The U.S. is making progress on two-thirds of the goals set in the Healthy People 2000 program to improve the nation's health. Positive trends: Americans are more active, using fewer drugs, riding in safer cars, testing their homes for radon and quitting cigarettes. But problem areas remain, including: homicide, nutrition, teen pregnancy, occupational injuries, chronic disease and pneumonia deaths."[8]

Reliastar Health Indicators The health indicators put together by Relia-Star Financial Corporation (formerly known as Northwestern National Life) are based on 17 factors. ReliaStar's rankings are widely recognized as the most comprehensive analysis of the relative health of the populations in all 50 states. The 17 indicators are as follows:

- lifestyle
    —prevalence of smoking
    —motor vehicle deaths
    —violent crime
    —risk for heart disease
    —high school graduation
- access
    —unemployment
    —adequacy of prenatal care
    —lack of access to primary care
    —support for public health care
- disability
    —occupational fatalities
    —work disability status
- disease
    —heart disease

—cancer cases
—infectious disease
* mortality
—total mortality
—infant mortality
—premature death[9]

Commitment to Public Service

Boards committed to community stewardship will also help bring resources to people in need; they will bring together the haves and the have nots. As The Healthcare Forum points out, "A healthier community is not something any single group—including those devoted to health care—can accomplish alone. The community has to do it. What health care organizations can do is to become catalysts—provoking changes far beyond our campuses calling forth energies far greater than our own."[10]

John McKnight and John Kretzmann, in their book *Building Communities from the Inside Out,* talk about the need to view hospitals as assets within the community. They describe a technique called mapping, in which health care organizations are linked with appropriate community partners. McKnight and Kretzmann see four sets of potential community partners for health care organizations:

* various kinds of community organizations and associations
* publicly funded institutions such as schools and the police
* business organizations, including small local businesses and branches of large corporations
* individuals and groups with special interests, abilities, and capacities, such as senior citizen and youth groups[11]

When governance teams serve the public, they become connected to their communities in new and meaningful ways. New partnerships and collaborations are formed to serve community interests.

Community Stewardship Case Examples

There are many examples of community stewardship in the United States, from small, local initiatives to national programs. Regardless of the scope of the initiative, health care organizations are forming partnerships with others to help their communities. The two examples of community stewardship that follow represent a movement committed to ending hunger and poverty and a grassroots effort to bring together thousands of volunteers to create change in the city of Atlanta.

World SHARE World SHARE, in San Diego, California, is an organization dedicated to the relief of hunger and poverty. It provides monthly food packages to more than 500,000 families in the United States, Mexico, and Guatemala every month, in exchange for a commitment to community service. Service may be contributing to the construction of a road, removing graffiti, establishing playgrounds, or distributing food. Several health care organizations have worked with World SHARE to create the volunteer pool to serve the community and improve its health status.

The Atlanta Project The Atlanta Project (TAP) assists people in inner-city communities. It focuses on children and families, education, housing, economic development, public safety, health, and the arts. Working with corporate, academic, and service provider partners, TAP has organized hundreds of programs. It focuses on teenage pregnancy, drop-out rates, juvenile delinquency, crime, homelessness, and unemployment. TAP works with corporations, other nonprofits, and universities.

VISIONARY LEADERSHIP

"In times of dynamic change, it is critical that boards have a solid commitment to what they want to be—their vision and mission."

The second core competency of highly successful boards is visionary leadership. A vision is a clear picture of the future that people strive to create. Warren Bennis and Burt Nanus in *Leaders: The Strategies of Taking Charge* state that "to choose a direction, a leader must first have developed a mental image of a possible and desirable future state of the organization. This image, which we call a vision, may be as vague as a dream or as precise as a goal or mission statement. A vision is a target that beckons."[12]

Ultimately, the board is charged with the responsibility of ensuring that the organization fulfills its mission and vision. Boards should therefore view statements of mission and vision as important tools for guiding their organizations toward the realization of community health. These statements should describe, in general terms, the purpose of the organization and the ends to which it aspires. In so doing, the statements inform the community about what the organization is and what promises it intends to fulfill. In addition to communicating the organization's identity to outsiders, the mission and vision statements help boards set priorities, make decisions, and evaluate progress toward meeting goals.

The Mission Statement

The effective board has a clear sense of mission on which all board members agree. A simple test of board consensus—a component of board effectiveness—is to ask each board member individually to write the organization's mission on a sheet of paper. Next, compare the mission statements. Effective boards will find that they are in agreement. Ineffective boards will find no clear mission or, worse yet, several conflicting missions. To be effective, the board must know its organization's fundamental purpose for being in business. A board that is devoted to building healthier communities will see this goal as part of its mission.

The Vision Statement

The organization's vision statement should link the organization to the community. The organizational vision and community vision should be inseparable. There are many steps that boards can take to create effective visions. For example, boards may try some of the following:

- See the vision in the present, and write the vision in the present tense, as if it were already realized.
- Develop a vision that is a stretch for the organization but nonetheless attainable.
- Ascertain what will matter most to the organization in the future.
- See the board as part of the vision. What will they be doing? How will it feel?
- Invite others to be part of the visioning process, and remember that smaller visions add up to a larger vision of a healthy community.

In addition, boards can choose from a variety of frameworks to monitor achievement of their vision. One of the most effective is that of St. Joseph's Mercy of Macomb. (See figure 4-2.) On a single piece of paper, the St. Joseph's Mercy governance team can effectively monitor its mission, strategic focus, objectives, indicators, means and methods, and actions. This tool can also be used to communicate the organization's strategic intent, thus creating effective alignment among all the constituents.

Visionary Leadership Case Examples

There are many excellent case examples of visionary leadership across the country. The three examples of visionary leadership that follow represent Disney's vision of a healthy community, Lifespan's vision, and The Manchester Agenda.

FIGURE 4-2. St. Joseph's Mercy of Macomb Strategic Plan

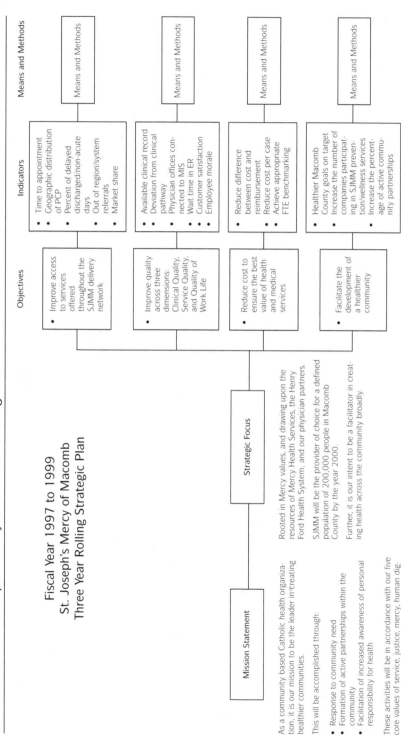

Fiscal Year 1997 to 1999
St. Joseph's Mercy of Macomb
Three Year Rolling Strategic Plan

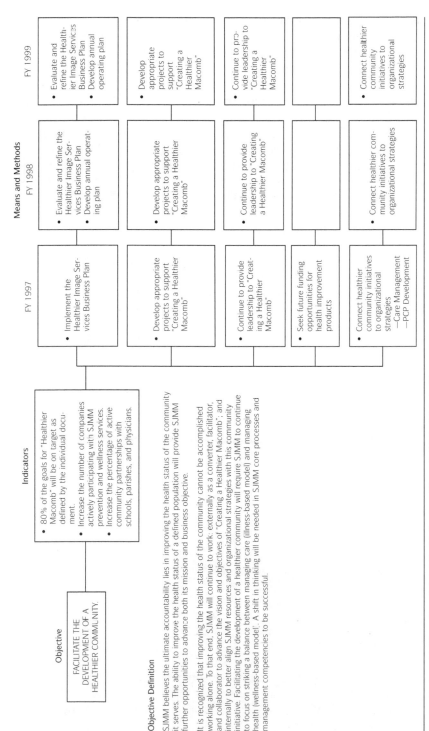

Means and Methods

Indicators	FY 1997	FY 1998	FY 1999
• 80% of the goals for "Healthier Macomb" will be on target as defined by the individual document. • Increase the number of companies actively participating with SJMM prevention and wellness services. • Increase the percentage of active community partnerships with schools, parishes, and physicians.	• Implement the Healthier Image Services Business Plan	• Evaluate and refine the Healthier Image Services Business Plan • Develop annual operating plan	• Evaluate and refine the Healthier Image Services Business Plan • Develop annual operating plan
	• Develop appropriate projects to support "Creating a Healthier Macomb"	• Develop appropriate projects to support "Creating a Healthier Macomb"	• Develop appropriate projects to support "Creating a Healthier Macomb"
	• Continue to provide leadership to "Creating a Healthier Macomb"	• Continue to provide leadership to "Creating a Healthier Macomb"	• Continue to provide leadership to "Creating a Healthier Macomb"
	• Seek future funding opportunities for health improvement products		
	• Connect healthier community initiatives to organizational strategies —Care Management —PCP Development	• Connect healthier community initiatives to organizational strategies	• Connect healthier community initiatives to organizational strategies

Objective

FACILITATE THE DEVELOPMENT OF A HEALTHIER COMMUNITY.

Objective Definition

SJMM believes the ultimate accountability lies in improving the health status of the community it serves. The ability to improve the health status of a defined population will provide SJMM further opportunities to advance both its mission and business objective.

It is recognized that improving the health status of the community cannot be accomplished working alone. To that end, SJMM will continue to work: externally as a converter, facilitator, and collaborator to advance the vision and objectives of "Creating a Healthier Macomb"; and internally to better align SJMM resources and organizational strategies with this community initiative. Facilitating the development of a healthier community will require SJMM to continue to focus on striking a balance between managing care (illness-based model) and managing health (wellness-based model). A shift in thinking will be needed in SJMM core processes and management competencies to be successful.

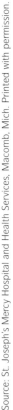

Source: St. Joseph's Mercy Hospital and Health Services, Macomb, Mich. Printed with permission.

Disney's Celebration Health When Disney, the entertainment and recreation conglomerate, decided to create a town called Celebration, Florida, it sought to move beyond the traditional concerns of real estate developers and to make a commitment to the education, health care, and quality-of-life concerns of its inhabitants. Because the company lacks expertise in health issues, it developed partnerships with organizations including Florida Hospital and the International Health Futures Network. Disney's vision is expansive: "Bits and pieces of what's being done [in Celebration] will be replicated in other communities, setting precedents for the way health care, education, and technology are integrated throughout communities in the future."[13] When a leader develops a mental image of what is possible, the results can be far reaching.

Lifespan Lifespan, in Providence, Rhode Island, is a large health system with total gross revenues of $742 million; 1,612 beds, including 1,374 general acute beds, 136 psychiatric beds, and 102 rehabilitation beds; 60,037 hospital admissions; 224,000 outpatient visits; 286,000 home care visits; and 38,419 outpatient surgeries. One Lifespan board member summed up Lifespan's philosophy as follows: "The community owns us; we don't own ourselves." The board's commitment to community health is reflected in the organization's statements of mission and key vision elements:

> The mission of Lifespan is to improve the health status of the people whom we serve in Rhode Island and southern New England through the provision of customer friendly, geographically accessible, and high value services. We believe this can best be accomplished within the environment of a comprehensive, integrated academic health system.
>
> Lifespan will be accomplishing its mission when it is recognized as
>
> 1. an organization that progressively strives to improve the health status of the community it serves
> 2. a geographically accessible, comprehensive, integrated health system
> 3. an organization that provides the highest value services, as demonstrated by its selection as the provider of choice for the majority of residents in its service area
> 4. an organization that works in productive partnership with physicians, other stakeholders, and suppliers
> 5. strongly committed to education and research in partnership with the Brown University School of Medicine and other allied health educational programs
> 6. a financially viable and a responsible steward of community resources.[14]

Lifespan actively seeks out a preferred future and creates its own path to achieve its vision. As such, it exemplifies visionary leadership.

The Manchester Agenda In 1993, thirty civic and business leaders gathered in Wolfeboro, New Hampshire, to develop a compelling shared vision of greater Manchester's future. Executives from both hospitals in Manchester, as well as several board members, participated in the two-day summit. Below are excerpts from the resulting vision statement:

> In the year 2000, Manchester, the "City with a Heart," is considered one of the top U.S. cities in which to live, play, and visit. People and companies are drawn to the greater Manchester area because it is an inviting, clean, and safe community.
>
> We are a diverse community known for our premium quality of life, an excellent education system and our educated workforce. We are proud of our history and our heritage. We are proud of our never-ending efforts to continually improve our community—including our recent economic revitalization. There is a strong sense of community identity and well-being. The basic needs of our people are being met through the availability of a wide range of quality housing, a well-supported, highly-regarded human service network, and an efficient, integrated health care delivery system. We are equally proud of our natural environment. We protect and utilize those resources—such as our river—with sensitivity and appreciation. . . .
>
> Our government structure has been revamped and strengthened. Elected officials see their role as setting policy and direction rather than micro-managing operations and services. It is mission-driven, innovative, and takes a long term focus. A clearly defined master plan has been developed, working with private sector groups and regional entities. Much of the bureaucracy has been eliminated; it is now experienced as "user-friendly" and responsive. Evaluation and improvement occur constantly.

The vision of Manchester in the year 2000 exemplifies an effective vision statement. It is positive, action-oriented, detailed, and inspirational.[15]

SYSTEMS THINKING

> "The issues facing boards today are so complex that we can't even begin to work through them until we learn how to think

systematically. We need a new set of skills to deal with this new wave of change. Our thinking in the future must be different."

Systems thinking is the third core competency of highly effective boards. Peter Senge defines system thinking as "a discipline for seeing wholes. It is a framework for seeing interrelationships rather than things, for seeing patterns of change rather than status snapshots."[16] Senge goes on to describe systems thinking as follows:

> A cloud masses, the sky darkens, leaves twist upward, and we know that it will rain. We also know that after the storm, the runoff will feed into groundwater miles away, and the sky will grow clear by tomorrow. All these events are distant in time and space, and yet are all connected within the same pattern. Each has an influence on the rest, an influence that is usually hidden from view. You can only contemplate the whole, not any individual part of the pattern. Business and other human endeavors are also systems. They, too, are bound by invisible fabrics of interrelated actions, which often take years to fully play out their effects on each other. Since we are part of that lacework ourselves, it's doubly hard to see the whole pattern of change. Instead, we tend to focus on snapshots of isolated parts of the system and wonder why our deepest problems never seem to get solved.[17]

Systems thinking is a way of looking at constellations of interacting parts and understanding how they function as a whole. If you want a large number of people to operate in a coordinated manner, they must share an image of the system of which they are a part. Applied to health care, systems thinking means seeing the health care organization as only one piece of the healthy community puzzle. More often than not, organizations deal only with their own piece of the puzzle. They make significant internal changes and modify relationships with others in the community without understanding the unintended consequences on community health. As we move into the 21st century, governance teams must stop seeing themselves as trustees of institutions and begin picturing themselves as governors of systems and relationships.

Six Systems Thinking Skills

Governance teams that understand how their organizations fit into the big picture share six skills of systems thinking: the ability to engage in public dialogue, collaboration, and a shared vision; and the ability to set strategic priorities, make use of common values, and participate in collective decision making.

Public Dialogue Public reflection refers to the ability to create common ground and build new shared assumptions. Many governance teams have found that community forums are helpful arenas for reflecting publicly on healthy community visions and progress made toward realizing these visions. Public dialogue in a community forum can help boards make the connections that might otherwise be overlooked.

Collaboration Our communities are like a mosaic made up of many different parts. When these parts come together and collaborate, the community is strengthened. By collaborating with others, boards can begin to understand interrelationships and patterns of behavior that may have eluded them in the past.

Shared Vision One board chair, in speaking about his organization's relationship to the community, said to me, "We are only one small part of our community's mosaic. My organization's vision is only one small part of the mosaic. A shared vision will allow us to see the pattern of the mosaic and not just our small strand." The ability to create a shared vision is a very important systems thinking skill.

Strategic Priorities Another important systems thinking skill is the ability to set strategic priorities that have an impact on the community system. For one health care organization, setting strategic priorities meant a different approach to the health problem of crack-addicted babies. Systems thinking helped the organization understand the interrelationship between environment and neonatal health. In the past, the organization would have seen only the separate event—the crack-addicted baby—but systems thinking allowed the organization to see the causes of the event. The health care organization wound up investing $250,000 in rehabilitating a two-block section of the neighborhood instead of investing the same amount in the hospital's neonatal intensive care unit. Thus, the intervention became a primary care intervention rather than a tertiary care intervention. As this example shows, strategic priorities change when health care organizations practice systems thinking.

Common Values Common values bring people in the community together and unite them in a common cause. Board members who listen to community members express their hopes and fears may be surprised by what they hear, but with dialogue and, perhaps, debate, both sides will discover common ground. It is important that consensus on vision and values be put in the context of community health decisions that will be made in the future. Rather than viewing the relationship between the organization and the community as a *struggle*, try finding a *balance*.

Collective Decision Making and Joint Accountability A final skill required for systems thinking is the ability to make decisions with the collective input of the stakeholders. A related skill is planning; a plan must be put in place so that results can be monitored and there is joint accountability for the results. When governance teams practice systems thinking, they discuss the goals of the organization in concert with community goals, rather than looking at their own organization and its desired outcome in isolation.

Integration of Services and Systems Thinking

Twenty-first-century governance will move from complication management to disease management and then to health management primarily through integration of services. Integration does not necessarily mean merger and consolidation, trends that have affected many health care organizations in the 1990s. Integration does mean, however, that strategic alliances and relationships will be formed in order to care more effectively for the health of a geographic region and gain certain competitive advantages. For example, strategic alliances typically improve the organization's cost advantage or provide some form of differentiation that the organization would otherwise be without.

A Service Integration Process One integration approach governance teams have taken is to integrate with others and design a system of care offering a continuum of services. This process involves five steps:

1. Identify existing and potential strategic alliances and relationships.
2. Assess the value of the strategic alliance and relationship.
3. Develop a draft vision of the integration strategy, statement of purpose, and operating principles.
4. Identify the structural arrangement that will accomplish the integration strategy.
5. Create the new strategic alliance and relationship and monitor its performance based on critical success factors.

To construct a list of possible strategic alliances and relationships, boards might identify the source of the relationships, their potential organizational forms, and the integration opportunity. (See table 4-2.) Potential alliance partners may include primary care physicians, payers, hospitals, and venture capital partners, to name only a few. The possible integration opportunity may include capital formation, information systems, and practice management. In short, governance teams need to construct possible scenarios for all potential strategic alliances and relationships and create the scenarios that are most likely to lead to the success of the health care organization. There are many models and structured ways to integrate services, ranging from loose to tight affiliations to "virtual mergers," in which the asset base is kept separate but revenue and expenses are shared, regardless of the site of care.

Two Approaches to Board Integration   Often, service integration is preceded by board integration. A range of opportunities exists to help our governance teams integrate effectively. Two models to consider are the strategic alliance model and the integrated system model. The strategic alliance model is a partnership of autonomous organizations for specified purposes. With this approach, both boards retain undiluted authority and autonomy. The alliance could be a primary but not an exclusive relationship, voluntary and renewable rather than permanent. In contrast, the integrated system model represents a parent-corporate relationship. With this approach, two independent organizations are united under one governance structure and executive leadership. Regardless of the approach to board integration, boards must draft an alliance or integrated system vision and provide strategic direction to guide the new arrangement so that they create a system that functions as a whole.

TABLE 4-2. Integration Scenarios

Source of the Relationship	*Potential strategic alliance partner(s)*	*Potential organization form*	*Integration opportunity*
Improved health status	Hospitals, business and industry, other nonprofits	Healthy community foundation	Capital, people, volunteers
Network development	Physicians, payers, primary care group	Management services organization	Information services, credentialing, practice management
Managed care contracting	Hospitals, physicians	Physician-hospital organization	Capital utilization management

Systems Thinking Case Examples

Many health care organizations have begun to practice systems think-ing. The Southcentral Health Network is a coalition focused on system-atic change. The Heart, Body and Soul Program represents a partnership of community organizations to improve the quality of life in east Baltimore. The California Healthy Cities Project focuses on the city and its total environment.

Southcentral Health Network The Southcentral Health Network in Idaho is a coalition of area hospitals, health agencies, and a commu-nity college. The vision of the network is a healthy southcentral Idaho in the year 2012 (the year that children born in 1994 will graduate from high school). The mission of the network is "to promote a cooperative effort of communities to improve the health of residents of South-central Idaho." To fulfill this mission, the coalition sponsored a com-munity health assessment, the goal of which was to identify the community's most critical health problems. The assessment process was adopted from the Assessment Protocol for Excellence in Public Health (APEXPH), a health planning model designed by the American Public Health Association, and from the Healthy Communities 2000 national initiative. The community health assessment had three parts: (1) an analysis of health information, (2) a community health needs survey, and (3) the selection of community health priorities. Analysis of community perceptions from the health needs survey, in conjunc-tion with an examination of health status data and availability of health services and programs and health-related policies, resulted in the network's prioritization of the community's health concerns. They are as follows:

1. alcohol and other drugs
2. cancer
3. heart disease
4. unintentional injuries
5. maternal and infant health

The next steps taken were to organize expert teams, assess com-munity resources, develop strategic and identifiable objectives, and solicit community-wide collaboration.[18]

The area hospitals that participated in this initiative understood that they must collaborate with others to improve the health of the com-munity's residents. One board member told me that the formation of the network "allowed us to think systematically and devote our full atten-tion and resources to the community health priorities and not to any one organization's priorities."

The Heart, Body and Soul Program The community of east Baltimore faces increasing morbidity and mortality rates, high unemployment, crime, substandard housing, and a deficient educational system. The Heart, Body and Soul Program unites community organizations, governmental agencies, businesses, and health care providers to address the health problems and to enhance the quality of life and well-being of the community.

The partnership's vision is to "strengthen collaborative efforts to revitalize and redevelop the east Baltimore community." It is concentrating on the areas that have been identified as priorities and that can be addressed most effectively: smoking, hypertension, diabetes, tuberculosis, cancer, violence, substandard housing, drug use, and coronary disease. Immunization and drug treatment programs are also in place. The Heart, Body and Soul Program has established prevention centers, a neighborhood health training program, community crime patrols, crime prevention education, housing development, educational programs, and economic development plans. In keeping with its stated goal of "community-ownership," the community not only indicates a preference for certain programs but also designs, conducts, and "owns" its programs.[19]

The California Healthy Cities Project The California Healthy Cities Project is part of a growing international public health movement that focuses on the city and its total environment—including the physical surroundings, economic conditions, and social climate—as an arena for health promotion activities. The project encourages public, private, and voluntary sectors to work in concert with community residents to identify and address health priorities and related issues of livability. The development of responsive public policies, which preserve and promote individuals and community health, is the key to the Healthy Cities approach.

Project participation begins with attendance at an orientation session and includes the successful completion of the following steps:

- passage of a city council resolution that endorses participation in the California Healthy Cities Project and reflects commitment to the Healthy Cities concept
- identification and recruitment of local steering committee members
- submission of a project application and work plan

While project participation usually begins with the design and implementation of a specific project, the process of creating a healthy city is expected to be an ongoing commitment to a collaborative, participatory style of governance.[20]

HIGH-LEVERAGE ACTIONS

"It's a lot easier to fly at 40,000 feet, scan the landscape, and begin with the big picture."

The fourth core competency of highly effective boards consists of three high-leverage actions: mastering change, practicing effective strategic planning, and communicating effectively. These actions enable governance teams to chart a future direction and ensure their organization's best chance of success.

Mastery of Change

Respondents to my 21st-century governance survey (appendix A) identified mastering change as the most important board skill. To effectively manage change, boards must understand how change occurs. Health care issues are complex; economic, demographic, scientific, and political forces affect them in ways that are sometimes unpredictable. The advent of managed care has raised the level of complexity and the rate of change. Mastery of the change process is an essential skill, and it is useful to analyze change as occurring in four stages.

Stage 1: Pressure to Change The first stage of the change process is feeling pressure to change. Pressure may be exerted by a variety of internal and external forces, such as regulatory pressure, competitive pressure, cost and financial performance, reform initiatives at the state and federal level, and technological changes. Consider the following examples:

- A health care system in the Southwest recognized the need to change, as a result of deregulation and the elimination of the certificate of need, which regulates the expansion of existing and new health care services over a certain dollar threshold. For-profit organizations offering alternatives to traditional inpatient and ambulatory care quickly moved into the state to capture the market. Managed care grew from 12 percent of the local market to 45 percent in less than one year.
- A small rural hospital in New England felt pressure to change as a result of managed care, a rapidly eroding financial base, and the loss of two key admitting physicians.
- A governance team in the South decided to sell to a for-profit organization after years of poor financial performance, loss of market share, and the inability to compete effectively with the other providers in the community.

The pressure to change typically occurs because of either a dissatisfaction in the level of an organization's performance or a competitive threat. Proactive boards, recognizing the pressure to change before it is too late, take appropriate action.

Stage 2: Vision to Change Proactive governance teams quickly move into stage 2 of the change process—imagining what the organization can become as a result of the pressure to change. During this stage, the board attempts to see a different image of its organization. Organizations that have gone through stage 2 include the following:

- A small acute care hospital in the Midwest, which decided to convert to primary and ambulatory care and affiliate with a large urban health care system. It created a different image of its future and got out of the inpatient business.
- A large health care system on the West Coast, which decided to acquire isolated hospitals and bring them into a managed care network. This move gave the large health care system a competitive advantage in its market.
- A loose alliance of hospitals and physicians on the East Coast that developed a new vision and implemented a health care system with tight integration of hospital and physician participation spread across a broad geographic market.

Each of these organizations had a proactive board that created a new vision for the organization and quickly reinvented itself to create solutions to problems.

Stage 3: Capacity to Change Capacity to change refers to the board's and organization's ability to manage change as well as change themselves. The capacity to change requires motivation and skill. It means commitment to achieving the new vision and enrolling others in the process to create alignment. In most cases, this is the stage in which the change process breaks down due to resistance. The success of the governance team will depend upon the board's motivation and ability to manage change. Organizations that have made it through stage 3 include the following:

- An acute care hospital in a small town in the Midwest faced a situation where the number of empty beds made the financial prospects dim. Some executives believed in the need to merge with another institution, but the community was resistant to such a merger. The board was able to enlist the support of prominent members of the community through dialogue and a commitment to retain the small-town character of the hospital.

- An inner-city emergency department was incurring unacceptable costs because members of the community were using the department for inappropriate purposes. When faced with the prospect of closing the emergency department, an alliance between the board and community leaders formed a program for education and preventive care.

As organizations develop and expand their capacities to change, the change process becomes more rapid, and the individual stakeholders grow more accustomed to change as an ever-present aspect of health care.

Stage 4: Plan for Change Managing complex change requires governance teams to have a clear but flexible action plan. This plan must include the resources required and time frames needed to realize the new vision. The change process is an iterative process. It creates recognizable successes. Change means the board must make choices in a highly volatile health care environment. When governance teams master change, they master their organization's destiny. Examples of organizations that have gone through stage 4, *plan for change,* include the following:

- An integrated care network in a major metropolitan area with a substantial market share in its region was acknowledged as a pioneer of responsible change in health care. The trustees had successfully led the drive to integrate, but rather than resting on their laurels, they started investigating alliances that would further their strategic plans, including a collaboration with the research facility of a medical school and the sponsorship of an initiative to educate young people at risk for AIDS.
- A health care facility in California with a strong physician staff responded to requests from within the community to incorporate alternative healing methods into its continuum of care. The board enlisted physicians in leadership roles to explore the possibility of collaborating with a center of holistic medicine and other local businesses and organizations.

Making plans for change involves taking stock of the organization in the context of the entire community and identifying ways to assess and revise existing change initiatives and to explore new challenges and initiatives.

Effective Strategic Planning

The second high-leverage action is to practice effective strategic planning. The success of any organization rides on the governance team's ability to plan strategically for its future. Strategic planning may be grouped into three components: the strategic planning process, the selection of strategic choices, and the implementation of the strategic plan.

The Strategic Planning Process   Ellen F. Goldman and Kevin C. Nolan, in *Strategic Planning in Health Care*, define strategic planning as "the process of strategy assessment, development, and implementation."[21] The decisions, actions, and evaluations during each of these three main steps correspond to the organization's culture and to the specific situations that are driving or inspiring the planning process. Strategic planning requires a sensitivity to the organization as well as a familiarity with the basics of the strategic planning process in any setting.

Looking at the overall health care field as well as the local health care market and the organization's position within the market, what is the picture? The strategic assessment includes health care market conditions and trends, the market's competitive structure, and future structural developments. Analyze the organization's operational and financial performance. Using a base-case financial scenario, assume that no significant changes are made and predict where you will be at some point in the future.

Strategy development includes evaluating alternative strategic directions for the operation. As a qualitative, process-oriented activity, strategy development requires creativity and scrutiny of the prevailing assumptions.

Selection of Strategic Choices   The second component of strategic planning is the selection among strategic choices and options. Every health care organization has strategic decisions and choices to make regarding its future. Some of the strategic choices and options mentioned most often by board chairs are listed below:

- *downsizing*—determining ways of reducing the expense of delivering health care services while retaining economic viability and an appropriate level of care
- *cost management*—seeking to provide health care services at the lowest possible cost in order to compete on a price basis
- *differentiation*—seeking to be unique along any number of its business lines
- *diversification*—moving into related health care activities so as to become less dependent on hospital revenues
- *market development*—gaining market share by strengthening referral networks, developing feeder systems, and developing preferred relationships
- *system development*—forming alliances of providers, payers, and managed care plans to develop continuum-of-care offerings

- *primary care development*—developing a base of primary care physicians that acts as a source of referrals and manages cost-effective care through a continuum
- *strategic alliances*—developing relationships with a range of providers, payers, business and industry, government, and community organizations to improve the health of the population and gain a strategic advantage
- *acquisition*—acquiring existing competing health care providers, programs, or services in order to compete more effectively
- *conversion*—converting existing capacity and resources to other related uses such as long-term care, home care, and subacute care
- *divestiture*—divesting existing facilities, programs, services based on profitability, market demand, and fit with organizational vision
- *quality*—providing high-quality services based on objective outcome research
- *merger or consolidation*—combining two or more health-related organizations to create a new legal identity
- *vertical integration*—developing a system of care with similar institutions providing coverage across an entire market
- *horizontal integration*—coordinating with such dissimilar providers as physicians, payers, and home care providers, to offer a range of services across a geographic region

Three governance tools can assist in planning. The first, the strategic governance grid, is a tool that the board can use to get a quick picture of what the organization's priorities are and whether they are short- or long-term and internally or externally focused. (See figure 4-3.)

The second useful tool is the governance priority matrix, which gives the board a snapshot of the organization's priorities, their stage of development on a project matrix, and their level of priority—high, medium, or low. (See table 4-3.)

The third tool is the governance quarterly assessment. (See table 4-4.) On a quarterly basis, the board is given a written status report of the organization's goals, key success factors, and a year-to-date assessment. One board member said to me that the three governance tools provided a "practical way of quickly monitoring existing or previous board actions and allows our board to spend more productive time strategically planning for our future."

Implementation of the Plan The third component of strategic planning is the implementation of the plan. This is the step during which an action plan is formed to identify the tasks to be accomplished, the roles and responsibilities of key players, and the timetable for each initiative in the plan. A well-wrought strategic plan can produce extraordinary performance by a health care organization.

FIGURE 4-3. Strategic Governance Grid

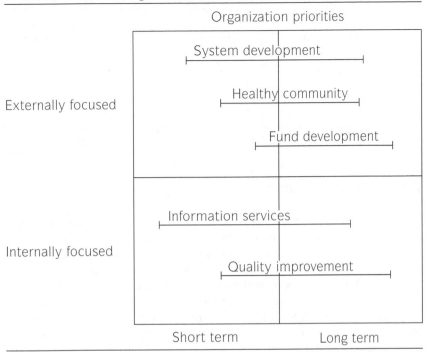

Organization priorities

Externally focused

- System development
- Healthy community
- Fund development

Internally focused

- Information services
- Quality improvement

Short term   Long term

TABLE 4-3. Governance Priority Matrix

	Project feasibility	*Project-planning status*	*Implementation schedule*	*Monitoring key indicators*
High priority— significant commitment of resources				
Medium priority— moderate commitment of resources				
Low priority— limited commitment of resources				

TABLE 4-4. Governance Quarterly Assessment

Organization goal	Key success factors	Year-to-date assessment
Financial viability	Key statistical and financial indicators	Status report
System development	Alliance, affiliation, physician alignment	Status report
Other goals	Key success factors	Status report

Effective Communication

In addition to mastering change and practicing effective strategic planning, boards must learn to communicate effectively. It is important to make explicit the governance process so that board members know what is expected of them. In addition, the effectiveness of the board is often determined by how well board members communicate with each other. The board must be willing to invest the time to examine how it communicates at board meetings and how it communicates the vision to a broader audience. The governance team is responsible for listening to the communities it serves and effectively communicating its future intentions.

The authors of *Getting to Yes* define four straightforward tips for effective communications under almost any circumstance:

• Separate the people from the problem.
• Focus on interests, not positions.
• Invent options for mutual gain.
• Insist on using objective criteria (in setting the terms of an agreement).[22]

Whether in the boardroom or in the community, when the board separates people from problems and focuses on common interests, it facilitates effective communication. Effective communication is a critical high-leverage action that leads to effective governance.

High-Leverage Actions Case Examples

Many health care organizations have taken high-leverage actions to gain a competitive advantage. The examples that follow illustrate how two organizations used the three high-leverage actions—mastering change, strategic planning, and effective communication—to chart different courses for themselves and for their communities.

St. Joseph's Mercy of Macomb St. Joseph's Mercy of Macomb, Clinton Township, Michigan, adopted a strategic planning system based on *hoshin* planning, "a planning and management system that focuses and aligns the organization to achieve breakthroughs for customers" in the words of Mara Minerva Melum and Casey Collett, authors of *Breakthrough Leadership.*[23] Inspired by the Japanese word *hoshin*, which means the needle of a compass, hoshin planning includes the following six elements:

- a focus for the organization
- a commitment to customers
- deployment of the organization's focus so that employees understand their specific contributions to it
- collective wisdom to develop the plan
- tools and techniques that make the hoshin planning process and the plan helpful, clear, and easy to use
- ongoing evaluation of progress to facilitate learning and continuous improvement

The St. Joseph's Mercy of Macomb Board planning committee met to revise the mission and vision of the organization. For two days, the board was educated on hoshin planning and the six key elements of hoshin planning. Board members also adopted four customer-focused objectives:

1. increased access to services offered throughout the St. Joseph's Mercy of Macomb delivery network
2. improved clinical quality, service quality, and quality of work life
3. reduced costs to ensure the best value of health and medical services
4. development of a healthier community

These four objectives remain constant, but the means and methods may change from year to year. To fulfill the fourth objective, *development of a healthier community,* the board's role was to revise the mission and vision, adopt the objectives, and monitor indicators on a monthly basis. (See figure 4-4.) Effective use of the high-leverage actions enabled St. Joseph's Mercy of Macomb to gain a competitive advantage and to create a healthier community.

Bethel New Life Since its founding 18 years ago, Bethel New Life has been at the forefront of efforts to revitalize Chicago's West Side. Bethel has gained a national reputation for cutting-edge initiatives and innovative approaches to economic development within its low-income, African-American community. As a community development corporation, Bethel embodies the belief that community-based initiatives must

FIGURE 4-4. St. Joseph's Mercy of Macomb Means and Methods

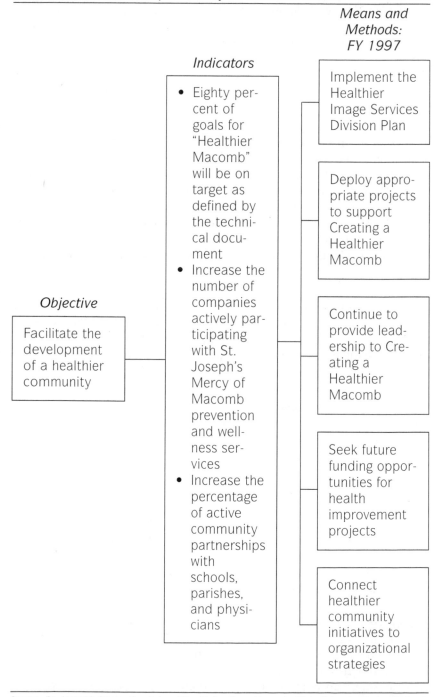

both lead and provide the foundation for any successful, enduring effort to create a healthier community.

Bethel takes a holistic and interdependent approach to community health, balancing spiritual leanings with clear economic, environmental, educational, and cultural objectives. It set out to develop economic security, environmental quality, and a high quality of life for all—a criterion measured by educational and employment opportunities, physical health, and personal safety.

Bethel took a leadership role in the West Garfield Park Empowerment Zone Collaborative, a coalition formed in response to the opportunity to be a part of a federally designated empowerment zone. A number of different partnerships joined together in this coalition. It focused on transportation, industrial and commercial development, housing redevelopment, education reform, family wellness, neighborhood safety, and health care.[24]

BASIC BUSINESS SKILLS

"As days per 1,000 continue to drop, and payments per patient continue to decline, only the creative, quality-oriented, cost-effective providers will survive."

Basic business skills are the fifth core competency of highly successful boards. There are three basic skills that will leverage boards to improve their organization's competitive position in the marketplace and provide them with a competitive advantage in both the short term and the long term: cost-effectiveness, quality improvement, and increased productivity. Adoption of these three basic skills will also lead to more cost-effective, integrated systems of care. A focus on these three skills is more important than a singular focus on any one of the basic skills. The chemistry of the three is best illustrated by what W. Edwards Deming describes as the "chain reaction." (See figure 4-5.)

Governance teams can readily see, from a systems perspective, that there is a crucial interaction among the three basic skills. According to the old paradigm of managing complications, these three basic skills would translate to downsizing, incremental improvements in care, and ratcheting down of human resources to do more with less. In the new paradigm of disease management, the basic skills translate to integration, managing care through pre- and posthospitalization, strategic relationships and alliances, improved health status, and retooling and retraining health care professionals. The role of the governance team is to foster an environment in which such new strategies can succeed.

FIGURE 4-5. The Deming "Chain Reaction"

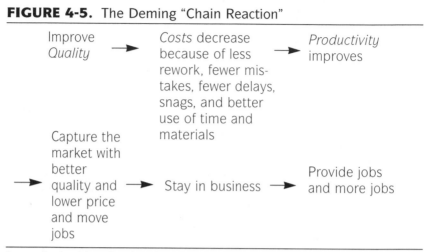

Source: Reprinted from *Out of the Crisis* by W. Edwards Deming; by permission of MIT and the W. Edwards Deming Institute. Published by MIT, Center for Advanced Educational Services, Cambridge, MA 02139. Copyright 1986 by the W. Edwards Deming Institute.

Cost-Effectiveness

The future survival of health care organizations will depend on how well they manage their costs. Governance teams need to recognize that cost-effectiveness will be the basis on which health care organizations compete throughout the age of managed care.

Characteristics of Cost-Effectiveness Board chairs from across the United States have shared with me their thoughts on cost-effectiveness. Certain key elements come up over and over again:

- financial viability as a component of the organization's vision statement
- a long-range financial planning process including a three-year financial forecast quantifying the level of financial performance needed to meet the long-term financial requirements of the health care organization
- a quarterly performance assessment of the goals, key success factors, and a year-to-date outlook. The latter should include the following:
  —net operating income
  —balance sheet and liquidity ratios
  —comparative cost and price position in the marketplace
  —achievement of targets consistent with A-rated health care organizations
- an ongoing operations improvement process that includes using a comparative database, identifying realistic opportunities, and following an operational improvement process to implement the change

- information systems that include cost accounting, decision support, and clinical case management
- benchmark indicators that are monitored using hospital operating indicators produced from data provided by Health Care Investment Analysts, Inc. (HCIA), of Baltimore, Maryland, and Standard and Poor's and Moody's ratios for A-rated organizations

A recent joint study by HCIA and Mercer Health Care Provider Consulting titled *100 Top Hospitals: Benchmarks for Success* establishes achievable, quantifiable performance measures that can be used by the industry as guidelines for improvement in an environment in which hospitals must work even harder at responding to market forces. The study concluded that if all of the nation's acute-care hospitals were to perform at the level of the 100 benchmark hospitals the following benefits would result: Nationwide expenses would decline by an aggregate 27 billion a year; the average lengths of stay would decrease by .88 days; and inpatient mortality would drop by 24 percent, and complications by 17 percent. In addition, profitability, growth in equity, and return on assets would increase significantly over current levels.[25] The results of the 1996 100 Top Hospitals study demonstrate the continued improvement of the health care industry. The results also indicate that further financial pressures lie ahead.

Actions That Lead to Cost-Effectiveness Governance teams that identify financial viability as part of their vision statement and that align the organization accordingly do get superior financial outcomes. Board chairs who commit to financial viability as a goal follow through with the following strategies:

- consolidation/merger
- strategic alliance
- elimination of unprofitable services
- integration of services
- consolidation of management
- reduction in scope of pursuits
- more aggressive management of costs
- "right-sizing"
- case management
- quality improvement focus with demonstrable improvements in clinical outcomes
- diversification of services
- priority on information systems

These strategies are aimed at more than just reducing costs; they also build the foundation for long-term fiscal stability.

Quality Improvement

The second basic skill is quality improvement. An organization's financial health and the level of quality it delivers are interrelated. When quality improves, costs go down. The governance role is to balance the economic discipline with a commitment to continuous improvement. Boards need to translate quality into practical governance terms; develop understandable benchmarks; and encourage the development of management, clinical, and community performance standards. It is important to understand three dimensions of quality:

- quality of the business practice
- quality of the care provided
- quality of the health status of the community

Quality of the Business Practice The board has ultimate responsibility for the quality of the business practice. The board establishes key business practice indicators with input from management. The board monitors how well the business practice functions are being carried out. One board chair said to me, "We monitor key financial indicators and ratios, but we go beyond that. We measure, through survey tools, the quality relationships we have with our patients, families, employees, physicians, business community, and our vendors. We provide quality patient care, which we measure. But we also measure the quality of our business practice quantitatively and qualitatively."

Quality of Care Provided The board also has ultimate authority and responsibility for the quality of care provided within the organization. Effective boards define the scope of the quality program, identify such critical success factors as clinical outcomes, and develop a way to monitor the quality of the care provided.

Quality of the Health Status of the Community Finally, enlightened boards, as part of their quality improvement, monitor and improve the quality of the health status of the community. Boards usually begin by noting the more common health status assessment indicators they need to monitor. A growing trend is the establishment of community quality councils that provide a forum to improve the quality of life in communities. Notable models of community quality councils exist in Pennsylvania, Wisconsin, Arkansas, and Connecticut. These community-based initiatives provide leaders of business, health care, education, and government an opportunity to share in the common goal of improving the health of the community.

Increased Productivity

The third basic skill is to increase productivity. Health care organizations and systems function as a collection of operating units and organizational processes—not just a collection of revenue and expense centers. To simply reduce costs without changing the basic clinical or business practice results in short-term cost savings. The role of the board is to support management in developing the three-year operations plan for the organization. The purpose of the operations plan is to increase productivity by improving operations and reducing costs simultaneously. Increased productivity translates to both a reduction in costs and an improvement in the clinical and business practice. The five elements of increased productivity are as follows:

- education of board and management
- assessment of the organization
- development of an effective benchmark
- identification and validation of opportunities
- development and monitoring of the three-year operations plan

Education of Board and Management Board education can take many forms, including individual research, group discussions, and visits with organizations and businesses from around the country. Management teams need a broad understanding of the cost structure of their organizational and system processes. An understanding of the federal and local environment helps in understanding the regulatory, fiscal, and health care reform pressures of the future. Board education also can mean participation in seminars and workshops with the boards from other organizations. In addition to the benefits of exchanging information and comparing strategies, board members may take comfort in finding out that many organizations are facing the pressures similar to the ones they face.

Assessment of the Organization To develop an effective three-year operations plan, it is critical that the organization know its current status in many respects. Key business and clinical indicators should be included as part of the organization assessment. The assessment should provide the board with baseline financial and clinical information that can be compared with that of other organizations.

Development of an Effective Benchmark The purpose of this step is to collect relevant comparative data and to construct a database to identify the four to six best-practice organizations. A board member may want to know how his or her organization compares with the best-practice organizations on business and clinical benchmarks. Or a member may want to consider best-practice opportunities that present themselves when two organizations consolidate.

Identification and Validation of Opportunities Once management has built the comparative database, it is the role of management to identify and validate the real opportunities for cost and process improvement. The board briefing should include an overview of the opportunities. Usually, successful benchmarking identifies short-term opportunities of one amount and long-term opportunities of another amount.

Development and Monitoring of the Three-Year Operations Plan The last element of increased productivity requires management to develop and implement the operations plan and prepare quarterly reports for the board. As with other board reports, key indicators are identified and monitored on a regular basis. Governance teams can effectively monitor how their health care organization or system is performing by using the governance benchmark profile. (See table 4-5.)

Boards of health care organizations have looked at operations in other industries to establish benchmarks. For example, they may look at the Ritz-Carlton Hotel Company for customer service, Walt Disney World for quality, or L. L. Bean for systems improvement. The governance benchmark profile provides a summary of the key issues concerning the board and lets it know how its organization is doing compared with other businesses both in and out of health care. The application of the three basic skills—cost-effectiveness, quality improvement, and increased productivity—will lead to an improved competitive position for the health care organization.

Basic Skills Case Examples

There are many excellent case examples of organizations that have improved their competitive positions through cost-effectiveness, quality

TABLE 4-5. Governance Benchmark Profile

Issue	Benchmark organization	Potential improvement	Time frame
Health status			
Operations			
Clinical management			
Consolidation			

improvement, and increased productivity. The first example is Hospital Corporation of America (HCA), now Columbia/HCA, one of the early pioneers in quality. The second case example represents a health care organization that went through a financial transformation and sustained its performance long term. The third example is outside of health care and represents an opportunity for a health care organization to benchmark and learn from others.

Hospital Corporation of America The Hospital Corporation of America in Nashville, Tennessee, began a quality improvement initiative in 1987. The initiative progressed gradually. First, a CEO and upper-level management of a hospital attended a session where they learned the basics of the quality outlook. Next, the HCA Quality Resource Group dispatched trainers to do on-site training in hospitals where the CEO agreed to teach part of the course. By 1990, HCA teams were at work on processes including billing, bed assignments, budgeting, and some clinical processes.[26]

Multiyear Restructuring at Stanford University Medical Center When Stanford University Medical Center completed its financial projections for 1990–91, it foresaw a $45 million loss. The reasons were twofold: its charges were relatively higher; and payer mix had changed, introducing a higher proportion of Medi-Cal patients. By overhauling its operations the medical center had progressed to the point where, by 1993, the board could forecast a surplus of a $26.6 million.[27] The multiyear restructuring effort at Stanford University Medical Center included improving quality, decreasing costs, and increasing productivity. The effort allowed the board members to leverage and improve their organization's competitive position in the marketplace.

The Ritz-Carlton Hotel Company The Ritz-Carlton Hotel Company in Boston, Massachusetts, is a leader in providing "the finest personal service and a quality product." The Ritz-Carlton's credo and the Ritz-Carlton basics are presented in figure 4-6. It is easy to appreciate how boards can learn from organizations outside health care. The practices at the Ritz-Carlton, if understood and adopted in health care organizations, could lead to increased quality and better relationships with patients and their families.

CONCLUSION

Our governance practices are being challenged, and the entire design of our institutions is being rethought. We are in the midst of leading systemic

FIGURE 4-6. Ritz-Carlton® Credo and Basics

Credo

The Ritz-Carlton Hotel is a place where the genuine care and comfort of our guests is our highest mission.

We pledge to provide the finest personal service and facilities for our guests who will always enjoy a warm, relaxed yet refined ambience.

The Ritz-Carlton experience enlivens the senses, instills well-being, and fulfills even the unexpressed wishes and needs of our guests.

The Ritz-Carlton® Basics

1. The Credo will be known, owned and energized by all employees.

2. Our motto is "We are Ladies and Gentlemen serving Ladies and Gentlemen." Practice teamwork and "lateral service" to create a positive work environment.

3. The three steps of service shall be practiced by all employees.

4. All employees will successfully complete Training Certification to ensure they understand how to perform to The Ritz-Carlton standards in their position.

5. Each employee will understand their work area and Hotel goals as established in each strategic plan.

6. All employees will know the needs of their internal and external customers (guests and employees) so that we may deliver the products and services they expect. Use guest preference pads to record specific needs.

7. Each employee will continuously identify defects through the Hotel.

8. Any employee who receives a customer complaint "owns" the complaint.

9. Instant guest pacification will be ensured by all. React quickly to correct the problem immediately. Follow-up with a telephone call within twenty minutes to verify the problem has been resolved to the customer's satisfaction. Do everything you possibly can to never lose a guest.

10. Guest incident action forms are used to record and communicate every incident of guest dissatisfaction. Every employee is

FIGURE 4-6. *(Continued)*

empowered to resolve the problem and to prevent a repeat occurrence.

11. Uncompromising levels of cleanliness are the responsibility of every employee.

12. "Smile—We are on stage." Always maintain positive eye contact. Use the proper vocabulary with our guests. (Use words like "Good Morning," "Certainly," "I'll be happy to" and "My pleasure").

13. Be an ambassador of your Hotel in and outside of the work place. Always talk positively. No negative comments.

14. Escort guests rather than pointing out directions to another area of the Hotel.

15. Be knowledgeable of Hotel information (hours of operation, etc.) to answer guest inquiries. Always recommend the Hotel's retail and food and beverage outlets prior to outside facilities.

16 Use proper telephone etiquette. Answer within three rings and with a "smile." When necessary, ask the caller, "May I place you on hold." Do not screen calls. Eliminate call transfers when possible.

17. Uniforms are to be immaculate. Wear proper and safe footwear (clean and polished) and your correct name tag. Take pride and care in your personal appearance (adhering to all grooming standards).

18. Ensure all employees know their roles during emergency situations and are aware of fire and life safety response processes.

19. Notify your supervisor immediately of hazards, injuries, equipment or assistance that you need. Practice energy conservation and proper maintenance and repair of Hotel property and equipment.

20. Protecting the assets of a Ritz-Carlton Hotel is the responsibility of every employee.

change; the five core competencies will allow our governance teams to deal with a constellation of interacting issues, not just the problems to be solved.

Highly effective boards begin with a sense of community steward-ship. Boards commit to the creation of healthy communities, and they focus on the health status of the population. With the guidance of their mission and vision statements, boards can exemplify the practice of visionary leadership. Once the ideals are in place, boards can start thinking about their organizations systematically and begin to see the connections to a much larger class of issues. Leadership demands high-leverage actions, which in times of rapid change in the industry include mastery of change, effective strategic planning, and effective communi-cation. The basic business skills are still important, and boards that concentrate on cost-effectiveness, quality improvement, and increased productivity will prepare their organizations to thrive in the 21st century.

References

1. Peter Block, *Stewardship: Choosing Service over Self-Interest* (San Francisco: Berrett-Koehler, 1993), p. 41.

2. John Immerwaher and Jean Johnson, *Second Opinions: Ameri-cans' Changing Views on Healthcare Reform* (New York: The Pub-lic Agenda Foundation, 1994).

3. Immerwaher and Johnson.

4. William Bowen, "Inside the Boardroom," *Princeton Alumni Weekly* (Feb. 22, 1995): 14.

5. The U.S. Department of Commerce, *Social Indicators III* (Wash-ington, D.C.: U.S. Department of Commerce, 1995), p. 2.

6. Richard Bayer and David Savageau, *Places Rated Almanac: Your Guide to Finding the Best Place to Live in America* (Chicago: Rand-McNally, 1997).

7. *The Prevention Index '89: A Report Card on the Nation's Health* (Emmaus, Pa.: Louis Harris and Associates, 1989).

8. "Strides Made Towards Goals of Wellness" *USA Today*, section D (Oct. 31, 1995).

9. Reliastar, *The ReliaStar State Health Rankings* (Minneapolis: Reliastar, 1995), p. 20.

10. The Healthcare Forum, *Healthier Communities Action Kit*, Mod-ule One (San Francisco: The Healthcare Forum, 1993), p. 3.

11. John McKnight and John Kretzmann, *Building Communities from the Inside Out: A Path toward Finding and Mobilizing a*

Community's Assets (Evanston, Ill.: Institute for Policy Research, Northwestern University, 1993), pp. 259–61.

12. Warren Bennis and Burt Nanus, *Leaders: The Strategies of Taking Care* (New York: Harper and Row, 1985), p. 89.

13. Shari Mycek, "A Clean Slate: Disney's Celebration of a Healthy Community," *Trustee* 48, no. 8 (Sept. 1995): 12.

14. Lifespan, *Vision, Mission, and Values* (Providence, R.I.: Lifespan, 1996).

15. Greater Manchester Chamber of Commerce, *The Manchester Agenda* (Manchester, N.H., 1993).

16. Peter Senge, *The Fifth Discipline: The Art and Practice of the Learning Organization* (New York: Doubleday/Currency, 1990), p. 6.

17. Senge, p. 68.

18. "The Southcentral Health Network of Idaho," in Richard Bogue and Claude H. Hall, Jr., eds. *Health Network Innovations: How 20 Communities Are Improving Their Systems through Collaboration* (Chicago: American Hospital Publishing, 1997), pp. 225–46.

19. The Heart, Body and Soul Program of East Baltimore, Clergy United for Renewal of East Baltimore (tel. 410/522-3430).

20. National Health Communities Initiative, *Healthy Communities Storybook* (Denver: National Civic League, 1992), p. 26.

21. Ellen F. Goldman and Kevin C. Nolan, *Strategic Planning in Health Care: A Guide for Board Members* (Chicago: American Hospital Publishing, 1994), pp. 23–24.

22. Roger Fisher and William Ury, *Getting to Yes: Negotiating Agreement without Giving In* (Boston: Houghton Mifflin, 1983), p. 11.

23. Mara Minerva Melum and Casey Collett, *Breakthrough Leadership: Achieving Organizational Alignment through Hoshin Planning* (Chicago: American Hospital Publishing, 1995), p. 16.

24. Bethel New Life, *Weaving a Healthy Sustainable Community* (Chicago: Bethel New Life, 1994).

25. Health Care Investment Analysts and Mercer Health Care Provider Consulting, *100 Top Hospitals: Benchmarks for Success* (Baltimore: HCIA, 1996).

26. Mary Walton, *Deming Management at Work* (New York: G. P. Putnam's Sons, 1990), pp. 85–86.

27. "Multi-Year Restructuring Changes Stick at Stanford University Medical Center," *Hospital Management Review* 12, no. 1 (Jan. 1993): 1.

Epilogue

Never doubt that a small group of thoughtful, committed people can change the world; indeed it is the only thing that ever has.

—*Margaret Mead*

The road to the future beckons us with opportunity. We are seeing the birth of a world economy, one in which cities and communities take on a new importance. In the 21st century, we will see regional collaboration and a renewal of community consciousness. To excel in the 21st century, boards must be willing to learn new skills. They must create environments conducive to learning; they must help their organizations value learning and change.

Peter Senge states in *The Fifth Discipline*, "Learning organizations are organizations where people continually expand their capacity to create the results they truly desire, where new and expansive patterns of thinking are nurtured, where creative aspiration is set free, and where people are continually learning how to learn together."[1] Governance teams that are building learning organizations are developing the capacity to work together. They are the leaders who are a step ahead of everyone else and who are leading systemic change in health care.

A NEW GOVERNANCE CULTURE

To make the transition to the new governance, governance teams must change their governance culture. They must examine the basic assumptions and beliefs that board members have learned by working together to adapt to the environment around them. The key is to realize that culture is learned and can only be understood in the context of the board's group process and its history. How boards lead, manage adversity, deal with environmental changes—these are all learned behaviors that have evolved over time. Because culture is learned, it can be changed. Boards can learn to build a new culture.

107

Below are two examples of organizations that challenged their deeply held beliefs and began to promote different behaviors at every level of the organization. In both cases, the community responded in a very positive manner. The first example is of a health care organization; the second, an inner city school.

From Competition to Collaboration

For a health care organization in an environment characterized by intense competition with a nearby hospital, the entire culture took on the competitive role. Not only was there a "corporate war" in the community, but this scenario played out at every level of the organization. Physician practices were acquired at the expense of the other hospital. There were two of every kind of technology, from magnetic resonance imaging equipment to helicopters.

A new CEO and a reconfigured board changed all that. A new vision, espousing collaboration, was presented to the organization and the community. A "eulogy" was held to say good-bye to the old beliefs. The board chair stated, "The old strategic plan served us well, but it is time to move away from the past." Over the course of 12 months, there were behavior changes at every level of the organization. The community's response was to embrace and support the change.

From Apathy to Action

An inner city school in the Midwest was in crisis. Students were dropping out of high school, and the school had some of the lowest test scores in the region. The city council became alarmed and brought in a new superintendent and principal. The first thing they discovered was that the deepest-held attitude by almost everyone in the school community was apathy. Simply stated, nobody cared. The new superintendent and principal decided to hold a funeral for Apathy at one of the large inner-city churches. The funeral was held and a sermon was given. Everyone had an opportunity to walk by an open casket, peer in, and say good-bye to his or her apathy. In the casket was a mirror. Students, teachers, and faculty were bidding farewell to their old selves. They were saying good-bye to their own deeply held beliefs. Over the course of 12 months, the school began to see a significant turnaround.

To change an organization's culture is not easy. Boards must say good-bye to a set of deeply held beliefs and attitudes. Declaration of a new culture does not bring one about, in and of itself. Deep cultural norms can only be changed by changing behavior. The board's behavior changes must be visible and experienced by both the community and the organization. A community collaborative is the organization's best opportunity to implement community initiatives or projects in conjunction with others interested in improving quality of life. It is an opportunity to develop new leadership and capitalize on the strengths of the community. It signals to the community that the board is serious about a new way of governing.

THE FOUR TYPES OF BOARDS

There are four distinct board types. In order to more effectively make the transition to the new governance, it is important to recognize your own board type. (See table 1.)

The Content Board

Content boards maintain the status quo. They tend to be reactive to the world around them. These boards play by the rules, and their organizations are principally operationally focused. Health care organizations led by content boards continue to do well through reengineering. However, the only way to create a long-term sustainable advantage is to be the best at playing by the rules. It gets very difficult for the content board to be successful when other boards are either changing or writing new rules.

TABLE 1. The Four Types of Boards

Content Board	Transitional Board	Progressive Board	Inventive Board
Maintain	Explore	Lead	Transform
Play by the rules	Confused by the rules	Change the rules	Write new rules
Operational	Strategic	Visionary	Inventive
Narrow definition of health	Moving toward a broader definition of health	Broad definition of health	Redefine health care
20th-century governance	20th-century governance	21st-century governance	21st-century governance

The Transitional Board

Transitional boards like to explore new possibilities and relationships. For the most part, they are confused by the rules. They have a tendency to play by some of the rules and not others. Some on the board like to hold on to the past while other board members can see a different future. The only way to create a long-term sustainable advantage for the organization is to quickly move to another stage of development—the progressive board.

The Progressive Board

Progressive boards like to lead and manage change to their advantage. The progressive board changes the rules to create a competitive advantage for its organization. These governance teams are politically astute and will build relationships that increase their size and capacity. They adopt a broad definition of health and practice many of the characteristics of 21st-century governance. They may create a health care system or a managed care company and begin to change old patterns and ways of doing things.

The Inventive Board

Inventive boards transform their organization by creating a new identity. These boards create fundamental change and seize upon new and different opportunities. These governance teams provide visionary leadership by inventing a fundamentally different concept of what could be.

THE GOVERNANCE PROFILE

Learning begins by understanding the current position of the organization. The governance profile—which appears as an appendix at the end of this epilogue—provides governance teams with a quick and easy assessment of their 21st-century governance competencies. This profile was developed at the request of several governance teams that expressed a desire to better understand and determine their own board's leadership gap. The governance profile is a tool that can be used to systematically measure a board's strengths and weaknesses by assessing the five core competencies of highly effective boards in the 21st century.

If our ability to learn is the only sustainable advantage, then the focus of the governance profile should be, not to rank boards, but to identify spots where the capacity to learn is inhibited. Once you have reviewed the governance profile, consider the action steps below in light of the results. The transition to 21st-century governance depends on self-reflection balanced with decisive action.

Following is a list of the statements from the governance profile organized by the five competencies, followed by recommended actions:

Community Stewardship: Related Statements from the Governance Profile

1. Our governance team has a broad sense of responsibility and commitment to serve our communities.
6. Our governance team recognizes that the real value of the board's power is to accomplish things that improve the health status of the community.
11. Our governance team consistently does what is in the best interest of the communities it serves.
16. Our governance team focuses on the health of the populations we serve.

Community Stewardship: Recommended Action

Governance teams should consider the following suggested action steps if the average column score for the community stewardship column falls below 16 points.

- A logical starting point for community stewardship is to better understand the community-building assets of the health care organization and to link these assets with appropriate partners in the community.
- Identify the critical determinants of a healthy community for the populations served by the health care organization.
- Define the organization's definition of health.
- Decide whether community stewardship, including the three important areas, comprises a key element of the organization's vision.
- Expand the board's tool kit to include a review and adoption of the health status indicators available today.
- Understand the relationship between the medical causes of death and lifestyle factors attributable to them.
- Working with others, conduct a health status assessment.
- Create one small success or adopt one initiative to gain some experience with community stewardship.

Visionary Leadership: Related Statements from the Governance Profile

2. Our governance team has collectively developed a clear mental image of a desirable future state for the organization.
7. Our governance team has a clear vision and mission that is broadly understood.
12. Our governance team has a high level of commitment to the vision and mission of the organization.
17. Our governance team is always proactive.

Visionary Leadership: Recommended Action

If the average governance team score for visionary leadership falls below 16 points, the governance team should consider the suggested action steps:

- Embark upon a visioning process that brings small visions together to create a whole context vision.
- After considering several scenarios for the organization's future, create a clear mental image of a desirable future.
- Develop a compelling organizational philosophy, purpose, and values. Remember that values put in context the decisions that will be made collectively as you move forward.
- Clearly communicate the vision internally and externally.
- If your definition of health embraces the concept of optimizing community health, then carefully think through how the care delivery system should be different.

Systems Thinking: Related Statements from the Governance Profile

3. Our governance team creates win-win situations, whether between two organizations or among several community organizations.
8. Our governance team has a primary goal to create strategic alliances and partnerships in order to more effectively care for the health of a geographic population.
13. Our governance team creates a learning environment that naturally leads to collaboration and cooperation internally and externally.
18. Our governance team recognizes patterns of change in the environment rather than individual events that affect the environment.

Systems Thinking: Recommended Action

Governance teams should consider the following action steps if the average column score for systems thinking falls below 16 points:

- Hold a healthy community forum that includes key constituents to identify issues systematically and to develop a community action plan.
- Discover common ground, understand the whole, and work with the community to develop a shared vision of the future.
- Identify systematically all of the potential relationships that exist today as well as those relationships that can potentially exist in the future. Assess the value of the relationship and develop coordinated integration strategies that create win-win situations.
- Create learning opportunities with community organizations and other groups your board has never talked to.
- Look for and create win-win situations with others in the community.

High-Leverage Actions: Related Statements from the Governance Profile

4. Our governance team has a set of clear priorities for the organization.
9. Our governance team effectively helps the organization adapt to change.
14. Our governance team has a multiyear plan to achieve the vision.
19. Our governance team clearly and effectively communicates with constituents and other organizations in the community.

High-Leverage Actions: Recommended Action

If the average governance team score for high-leverage actions falls below 16, the governance team should consider the following action steps:

- Conduct an assessment of where the organization is today. That should include an environmental, industry, organizational, and competitive assessment.
- Assess whether there is a compelling business reason to change.
- Develop a shared vision involving key stakeholders and prepare a transition plan that moves the organization forward from current reality to the new shared vision.

- Initiate a strategic planning process and select the strategic option that best positions the organization for the future.
- Develop a clear set of ground rules for how the board will conduct itself.

Basic Business Skills: Related Statements from the Governance Profile

5. Our governance team consistently demonstrates the organization's high-quality results through clinical outcomes and managing the course of disease proactively.
10. Our governance team consistently demonstrates that it is positioned as a cost-effective provider of care.
15. Our governance team recognizes that the strength of our organization is its ability to monitor and control costs.
20. Our governance team positions the organization to be a high-quality, cost-effective leader that has led to a sustainable advantage.

Basic Business Skills: Recommended Action

Governance teams should consider the following action steps if the average column score for basic business skills falls below 16 points.

- Include financial viability and quality improvement as a key element of the organization's vision statement.
- Develop a long-range financial planning process that meets the long-term financial requirements of the organization.
- Benchmark with other health care organizations.
- Expect from management a quality performance assessment of the organization's goals and key success factors.

The governance profile is a critical step in creating a highly successful board in the 21st century. Once the board has an assessment or profile of its 21st-century governance skills, it is easier to chart a future course.

Reference

1. Peter Senge, *The Fifth Discipline: The Art and Practice of the Learning Organization* (New York: Doubleday/Currency, 1980), p. 3.

The Governance Profile

Statements

Read each statement below and consider how it applies to you and your board, then circle the appropriate letter using the governance profile response form that follows the profile.

1. Our governance team has a broad sense of responsibility and commitment to serve our communities.

2. Our governance team has collectively developed a clear mental image of a desirable future state for the organization.

3. Our governance team creates win-win situations, whether between two organizations or among several community organizations.

4. Our governance team has a set of clear priorities for the organization.

5. Our governance team consistently demonstrates the organization's high-quality results through clinical outcomes and managing the course of disease proactively.

6. Our governance team recognizes that the real value of the board's power is to accomplish things that improve the health status of the community.

7. Our governance team has a clear vision and mission that is broadly communicated and understood.

8. Our governance team has a primary goal to create strategic alliances and partnerships in order to more effectively care for the health of a geographic population.

9. Our governance team effectively helps the organization adapt to change.

10. Our governance team consistently demonstrates that it is positioned as a cost-effective provider of care.

11. Our governance team consistently does what is in the best interest of the communities it serves.

12. Our governance team has a high level of commitment to the vision and mission of the organization.

13. Our governance team creates a learning environment that naturally leads to collaboration and cooperation internally and externally.

14. Our governance team has a multiyear plan to achieve the vision.

15. Our governance team recognizes that the strength of our organization is its ability to monitor and control costs.

16. Our governance team focuses on the health of the populations we serve.

17. Our governance team is always proactive.

18. Our governance team recognizes patterns of change in the environment rather than individual events that affect the environment.

19. Our governance team clearly and effectively communicates with constituents and other organizations in the community.

The Governance Profile *(Continued)*

20. Our governance team positions the organization to be a high-quality, cost-effective leader that has led to a sustainable advantage.

The Governance Profile Response Form

Respond to the questions in the space below; refer to the following key:

C = completely true   L = a little true
M = mostly true   N = not at all true
S = somewhat true

1	2	3	4
C M S L N	C M S L N	C M S L N	C M S L N
5	6	7	8
C M S L N	C M S L N	C M S L N	C M S L N
9	10	11	12
C M S L N	C M S L N	C M S L N	C M S L N
13	14	15	16
C M S L N	C M S L N	C M S L N	C M S L N
17	18	19	20
C M S L N	C M S L N	C M S L N	C M S L N

The Governance Profile *(Continued)*

Scoring

1. Circle the corresponding letter and number from the response form.
2. Total the columns.
3. Interpret the total score using the guide at the end of the appendix.

	Stewardship	*Visionary leadership*	*Systems thinking*	*High-leverage actions*	*Basic business skills*
	1 C 5 M 4 S 3 L 2 N 1	2 C 5 M 4 S 3 L 2 N 1	3 C 5 M 4 S 3 L 2 N 1	4 C 5 M 4 S 3 L 2 N 1	5 C 5 M 4 S 3 L 2 N 1
	6 C 5 M 4 S 3 L 2 N 1	7 C 5 M 4 S 3 L 2 N 1	8 C 5 M 4 S 3 L 2 N 1	9 C 5 M 4 S 3 L 2 N 1	10 C 5 M 4 S 3 L 2 N 1
	11 C 5 M 4 S 3 L 2 N 1	12 C 5 M 4 S 3 L 2 N 1	13 C 5 M 4 S 3 L 2 N 1	14 C 5 M 4 S 3 L 2 N 1	15 C 5 M 4 S 3 L 2 N 1
	16 C 5 M 4 S 3 L 2 N 1	17 C 5 M 4 S 3 L 2 N 1	18 C 5 M 4 S 3 L 2 N 1	19 C 5 M 4 S 3 L 2 N 1	20 C 5 M 4 S 3 L 2 N 1
Totals Grand total					

The Governance Profile *(Continued)*

Interpretation of the Governance Profile Score

The Governance Profile includes twenty items addressing a specific competency. The interpretation follows:

Governance teams in the *very effective* range (85–100) foster an environment that encourages community stewardship. Such teams have a clear and compelling mental image of where the organization wants to be. These teams respond to unanticipated changes and deal well with ambiguity. They have the capacity to work extremely well with many constituents. This governance team is a high-performing team and will be successful in the 21st century.

Governance teams in the *effective* range (71–85) generally are responsive to the communities they serve. They usually have clarity around the major elements of the organization's vision. They deal well with change and are able to change directions given the circumstances. They use high-leverage actions and the basic business skills to create a strategic advantage.

Governance teams in the *somewhat effective* range (56–70) may have difficulty gaining clarity around the organization's vision. They may serve the community on a programmatic basis but do not think of community stewardship as a fundamental value of the organization. These governance teams may react more to events and crises in the environment. These teams may respond to change, but the uncertainty can be troublesome.

Governance in the *ineffective* range (41–55) have problems gaining clarity around the organization's vision. Community service becomes secondary to putting out the fires. Sticking with the status quo and using strategies that worked well in the past seem to be the norm for these teams. Change occurs slowly, and oftentimes opportunities are missed.

Governance teams in the *very ineffective* range generally lack a vision and do not respond to unanticipated changes in the environment. Survival is the highest priority. These governance teams are not positioned favorably for 21st-century governance.

Appendix A
Competencies of Highly Successful Boards

THE RESEARCH METHODOLOGY

In 1994 I received the Governance Fellowship Award sponsored by the Governance Institute, La Jolla, California, and *Modern Healthcare*. The Fellowship Award funds research of timely or controversial governance issues. The research report I completed is entitled "21st Century Governance: Competencies of Highly Successful Boards." A national survey was sent to 3,800 board chairs of health care organizations in the United States. The survey grew out of discussions with trustees across the country about two topics: how 21st-century governance will be different and that a governance leadership gap may, in fact, exist. The health care survey that was sent to the 3,800 board chairs is shown in figure 1. The research revolves around two simple questions:

- What core leadership skills, capabilities, and values do trustees currently practice in their health care organizations?
- What core leadership skills, capabilities, and values will trustees need to practice in order to lead in the 21st century?

Thirty-one categories were rated on a scale of 1 to 5, with 1 being less important and 5 being critically important. Board chairs were also given the opportunity to add to the list of categories.

In addition, the board chairs were also asked to answer the following questions:

- How many beds does your organization have?
- Are you part of a health care system?
- What is your affiliation?
- If you had any advice for other board members, what would it be?

119

FIGURE 1. Governance Health Care Survey

Question 1: What core leadership skills, capabilities, and values do trustees currently practice in their health care organizations?

Question 2: What core leadership skills, capabilities, and values will trustees need to practice in order to lead in the 21st century?

Please indicate your response using the following rankings:
1 — less important
2 — somewhat important
3 — important
4 — very important
5 — critically important

Categories	Question 1. Current Practice	Question 2. Future Practice
1. Negotiation skills	1__ 2__ 3__ 4__ 5__	1__ 2__ 3__ 4__ 5__
2. Maximizing profits	1__ 2__ 3__ 4__ 5__	1__ 2__ 3__ 4__ 5__
3. Mastering change	1__ 2__ 3__ 4__ 5__	1__ 2__ 3__ 4__ 5__
4. Collaboration and cooperation	1__ 2__ 3__ 4__ 5__	1__ 2__ 3__ 4__ 5__
5. Management oversight	1__ 2__ 3__ 4__ 5__	1__ 2__ 3__ 4__ 5__
6. Accountability for broad geographic population	1__ 2__ 3__ 4__ 5__	1__ 2__ 3__ 4__ 5__
7. Visionary leadership	1__ 2__ 3__ 4__ 5__	1__ 2__ 3__ 4__ 5__
8. Community stewardship	1__ 2__ 3__ 4__ 5__	1__ 2__ 3__ 4__ 5__
9. Dominating the market	1__ 2__ 3__ 4__ 5__	1__ 2__ 3__ 4__ 5__
10. Increasing productivity	1__ 2__ 3__ 4__ 5__	1__ 2__ 3__ 4__ 5__
11. Focusing on health status of population	1__ 2__ 3__ 4__ 5__	1__ 2__ 3__ 4__ 5__

FIGURE 1. *(Continued)*

Categories	Question 1. Current Practice	Question 2. Future Practice
12. Systems thinking	1__ 2__ 3__ 4__ 5__	1__ 2__ 3__ 4__ 5__
13. Focusing on unmet health care needs	1__ 2__ 3__ 4__ 5__	1__ 2__ 3__ 4__ 5__
14. Empowering the community	1__ 2__ 3__ 4__ 5__	1__ 2__ 3__ 4__ 5__
15. Community health	1__ 2__ 3__ 4__ 5__	1__ 2__ 3__ 4__ 5__
16. Personal mastery	1__ 2__ 3__ 4__ 5__	1__ 2__ 3__ 4__ 5__
17. Team learning	1__ 2__ 3__ 4__ 5__	1__ 2__ 3__ 4__ 5__
18. Serving the public	1__ 2__ 3__ 4__ 5__	1__ 2__ 3__ 4__ 5__
19. Redefining health care	1__ 2__ 3__ 4__ 5__	1__ 2__ 3__ 4__ 5__
20. Communication skills	1__ 2__ 3__ 4__ 5__	1__ 2__ 3__ 4__ 5__
21. Mastering change	1__ 2__ 3__ 4__ 5__	1__ 2__ 3__ 4__ 5__
22. Relationships with constituents	1__ 2__ 3__ 4__ 5__	1__ 2__ 3__ 4__ 5__
23. Risk taking	1__ 2__ 3__ 4__ 5__	1__ 2__ 3__ 4__ 5__
24. Creating a healthy community	1__ 2__ 3__ 4__ 5__	1__ 2__ 3__ 4__ 5__
25. Strategic planning	1__ 2__ 3__ 4__ 5__	1__ 2__ 3__ 4__ 5__
26. Local accountability	1__ 2__ 3__ 4__ 5__	1__ 2__ 3__ 4__ 5__
27. Quality improvement	1__ 2__ 3__ 4__ 5__	1__ 2__ 3__ 4__ 5__
28. Cost effectiveness	1__ 2__ 3__ 4__ 5__	1__ 2__ 3__ 4__ 5__
29. Benchmarking	1__ 2__ 3__ 4__ 5__	1__ 2__ 3__ 4__ 5__
30. Integrating services	1__ 2__ 3__ 4__ 5__	1__ 2__ 3__ 4__ 5__

(Continued on next page)

FIGURE 1. *(Continued)*

Categories	Question 1. *Current Practice*	Question 2. *Future Practice*
31. Marketing	1__ 2__ 3__ 4__ 5__	1__ 2__ 3__ 4__ 5__
32. Others (please list) _____ _____ _____ _____	1__ 2__ 3__ 4__ 5__ 1__ 2__ 3__ 4__ 5__ 1__ 2__ 3__ 4__ 5__ 1__ 2__ 3__ 4__ 5__	1__ 2__ 3__ 4__ 5__ 1__ 2__ 3__ 4__ 5__ 1__ 2__ 3__ 4__ 5__ 1__ 2__ 3__ 4__ 5__

Please answer the following questions:

1. How many beds does your organization have? _____

2. Are you part of a health care system? Yes _____ No _____

3. What is your affiliation? Not for Profit _____ For Profit _____

    Governmental _____

4. If you had any advice for other board members, what would it be?

    _____

    _____

5. Comments:

    _____

    _____

Responses came from 655 board chairs across the United States, a 17 percent response rate. Of the 655 responses, 498 represented not-for-profit hospitals or systems, 81 were from for-profit organizations, and 76 were from governmental organizations. In addition to the survey responses, I also received 50 pages of advice from board chairs, directed to other board members across the country.

MAJOR RESEARCH FINDINGS

The research indicated that a significant leadership gap exists between our current governance practices and the skills and practices that board members will need to ensure the success of their organizations in the 21st century. Many of the board chairs intuitively sensed this gap after completing the survey. Fifteen core competencies of highly successful boards in the 21st century were identified by the 655 board chairs. Table 1 lists the not-for-profit and governmental board chairs' rankings of all the competencies currently practiced in the boardroom and compares them to their predictions of what the competencies of highly successful boards will be in the future.

While the two lists are similar, the research emphatically shows that significant statistical differences exist between the priorities and the relative weight the board chairs gave to each competency area. An interesting finding of the research is that the most significant gap between current practice and future practice exists in five key areas:

1. focusing on the health status of the population
2. systems thinking
3. creating a healthy community
4. redefining health care
5. integrating services

Table 2 lists the 15 competencies with the greatest discrepancy in ranking between current and future practice.

An incredibly interesting finding is that the first four practices listed above are not among the 15 core competencies used by board members today. More important, the areas showing the largest gap are related to the governance team's role in creating healthy communities, systems thinking, and redefining health care. In effect, board chairs are stating that health care organizations must take a greater role in creating health and must move away from individual-based sick care. Today's managed care/capitated environment creates a compelling business reason to focus on the health status of the population we serve. Board chairs have

TABLE 1. Governance Health Care Survey: Not-for-Profit and Governmental Rankings for all Competency Areas

Current Practice	Mean	Future Practice	Mean
15 Core Competencies of Highly Successful Boards			
Strategic planning	3.84	Mastering change	4.62
Quality improvement	3.83	Cost effectiveness	4.51
Cost effectiveness	3.83	Collaboration and cooperation	4.50
Mastering change	3.75	Visionary leadership	4.48
Visionary leadership	3.75	Strategic planning	4.43
Community stewardship	3.64	Quality improvement	4.28
Collaboration and cooperation	3.63	Integrating services	4.24
Management oversight	3.63	Community stewardship	4.16
Serving the public	3.61	Systems thinking	4.14
Communication skills	3.59	Communication skills	4.13
Maximizing profits	3.53	Creating a healthy community	4.13
Local accountability	3.47	Redefining health care	4.12
Increasing productivity	3.46	Focusing on health status of population	4.11
Relationships with constituents	3.35	Increasing productivity	4.11
Integrating services	3.27	Serving the public	4.06
Rankings for All Other Competency Areas			
Marketing	3.25	Risk taking	3.98
Redefining health care	3.13	Focusing on unmet health care needs	3.96
Focusing on unmet health care needs	3.12	Relationships with constituents	3.96
Creating a healthy community	3.12	Community health	3.93
Risk taking	3.09	Local accountability	3.92
Systems thinking	3.09	Maximizing profits	3.91
Team learning	3.07	Management oversight	3.85
Benchmarking	3.05	Benchmarking	3.79
Community health	3.01	Team learning	3.79
Focusing on health status of population	2.97	Marketing	3.76
Dominating the market	2.94	Accountability for broad geographic population	3.72
Personal mastery	2.88	Negotiation skills	3.55
Accountability for broad geographic population	2.88	Empowering the community	3.46
Negotiation skills	2.82	Dominating the market	3.26
Empowering community	2.72	Personal mastery	3.26

TABLE 2. Core Competencies: Greatest Mean Variations between Current and Future Practice

Current Practice— Mean	Categories	Future Practice— Mean	Gap, in Points	Gap, in Percentage
3.75	Mastering change	4.62	.87	23.2%
3.83	Cost-effectiveness	4.51	.68	17.8%
3.63	Collaboration and cooperation	4.50	.87	24.0%
3.75	Visionary leadership	4.48	.73	19.5%
3.84	Strategic planning	4.43	.59	15.4%
3.83	Quality improvement	4.28	.45	11.8%
3.27	Integrating services	4.24	.97	29.7%
3.64	Community stewardship	4.16	.52	14.3%
3.09	Systems thinking	4.14	1.05	34.0%
3.59	Communication skills	4.13	.54	15.0%
3.12	Creating a healthy community	4.13	1.01	32.4%
3.13	Redefining health care	4.12	.99	31.6%
2.97	Focusing on health status of the population	4.11	1.14	38.4%
3.46	Increasing productivity	4.11	.65	18.9%
3.61	Serving the public	4.06	.45	12.5%

indicated that this focus will be critical in the 21st century. Only those governance teams that choose to practice these 21st-century governance competencies will be highly effective in the future.

Twenty-first century governance will create new realities by concentrating on five important skill areas. When reviewing the 15 core competencies of highly successful boards in the 21st century, five natural groupings or clusters emerge. These groupings are listed in figure 2.

A WORD ABOUT FOR-PROFIT HEALTH CARE ORGANIZATIONS

The 81 board chairs of for-profit health care organizations indicated a set of competencies for 21st-century governance that is slightly different from that of the board chairs of not-for-profit and governmental organizations. (The 15 future competencies named by the for-profit board chairs are listed in table 3.) This variation does not mean that one list is necessarily more accurate than the other. We should attempt to understand the differences and recognize that this variance could be a learning opportunity for both for-profit and not-for-profit governance teams.

FIGURE 2. The Five Core Competencies of 21st-Century Governance

1. Community Stewardship
   - Creating healthy communities
   - Focusing on the health status of the population
   - Serving the public

2. Visionary Leadership
   - Redefining health care

3. Systems Thinking
   - Integrating services
   - Collaboration and cooperation

4. High-Leverage Actions
   - Mastering change
   - Strategic planning
   - Communication

5. Basic Skills
   - Cost-effectiveness
   - Quality improvement
   - Increasing productivity

While many of the competencies are similar, missing from the for-profits' top 15 competencies are serving the public, creating healthier communities, community stewardship, and focusing on the health status of the population. The for-profit list includes 4 competencies that are not in the top 15 competencies of the not-for-profit and governmental list:

- maximizing profits
- risk taking
- marketing
- relationships with constituents

Although profitability, in response to stockholder expectations, may be a higher priority for the for-profits, there are competencies, at the governance level, which the for-profits and not-for-profits share. One way of improving the health of our own organizations would be to establish a governance learning forum, in which for-profit and not-for-profit governance teams could benefit from the experience of others. Instead of judging each other on the basis of our priorities, we should realize that the real opportunity lies in our ability to improve the health of the nation by creating governance teams that can learn from each other.

TABLE 3. The 15 Future Competencies of For-Profit
Health Care Organizations

Future Practice	Mean
Mastering change	4.54
Cost-effectiveness	4.51
Visionary leadership	4.44
Collaboration and cooperation	4.40
Strategic planning	4.33
Integrating services	4.29
Quality improvement	4.23
Maximizing profits	4.22
Communication skills	4.15
Increasing productivity	4.09
Risk taking	4.06
Systems thinking	3.94
Marketing	3.87
Relationship with constituents	3.86
Redefining health care	3.85

Appendix B
Healthy Community Contract

We believe in the following fundamental truths:

- The quality-of-life issues facing our cities and communities can be identified and improved through a collaborative process that will lead to effective, long-term, sustainable solutions.
- Committed individuals along with other stakeholders in the community can effectively improve the health of its inhabitants.
- Health must be defined in its broadest sense and include such items as employment, safety, the environment, the economy, quality medical care, housing, diversity, and the meeting of basic needs.
- Our communities and cities can create global learning opportunities so that best practice interventions can be developed and shared worldwide.

Accordingly, we declare the following:

1. Our health care organization believes that the path leading to healthy communities and effective governance will converge in the 21st century.
2. We will adopt the three building blocks that lay the foundation for 21st-century governance. These are
   - the five principles of contemporary governance
   - the six-step process for creating and building healthy communities
   - the five core competencies of highly effective boards
3. We will collaborate and create partnerships with others to improve the health of our communities and adopt one of the three frameworks for creating healthy communities.

- The VHA Voluntary Community Benefits Standards: A Framework for Meeting Community Needs
- The Catholic Health Association Standards for Community Benefit
- The Hospital Community Benefits Standards Program

4. We will create an environment that focuses on community health, breaks down barriers, empowers the community, and allows us to design a healthy community.
5. We will understand the unmet health needs of the community and work together to fill the gap.
6. We will create and maintain a healthy organization that provides high-quality care in the most cost-effective manner.

Adopted _____

Board of Directors _____

Bibliography

The following bibliography is intended to help the reader interested in learning more about the topics covered in this book. The entries are grouped according to the five principles of 21st-century governance.

COMMUNITY STEWARDSHIP

American Public Health Association. *Healthy Communities 2000: Model Standards: Guidelines for Community Attainment of the Year 2000 National Health Objectives.* Washington, D.C.: American Public Health Association, 1991.

Block, Peter. *Stewardship: Choosing Service over Self-Interest.* San Francisco: Berrett-Koehler, 1993.

Breckon, D. J., J. R. Harvey, and R. B. Lancaster. *Community Health Education: Settings, Roles, and Skills for the 21st Century.* Gaithersburg, Md.: Aspen, 1994.

Catholic Health Association. *Reviewing the Catholic Healthcare Ministry: A Workbook in Community Accountability.* St. Louis, Mo.: Catholic Health Association, 1995.

Coile, Russell C. "Healthy Communities: Reducing Need (and Costs) by Promoting Health." *Hospital Strategy Report* 6, no. 4 (1984): 1, 3–5.

Elder, W. G., and B. A. Amundson. "The WAMI Rural Hospital Project. Part 3: Building Healthcare Leadership in Rural Communities." *Journal of Rural Health* 7, no. 5 (1991): 511–25.

English, J. C., and B. C. Hicks. "A Systems-in-Transition Paradigm for Healthy Communities." *Canadian Journal of Public Health* 83, no. 1 (1992): 61–65.

Ewell, C. M., and D. D. Pointer. *Really Governing: How Health System and Hospital Boards Can Make More of a Difference.* Albany, N.Y.: Delmar, 1994.

Hancock, T. "Developing Healthy Communities. A Five Year Project Report from the Community Health Development Centre. Presented at the International Healthy Cities Conference, September, 1994." *Canadian Journal of Public Health* 79, no. 6 (1988): 46–49.

Hancock, T., and L. Duhl. *Promoting Health in the Urban Context.* WHO Healthy Cities Paper No. 1. Copenhagen: FADL, 1988.

Hospital Research and Education Trust. *Background and Resources for a Community Health Status Focus.* Chicago: Hospital Research and Education Trust, 1994.

Hospital Research and Education Trust. *Trustees and the Integration of Community Health Care.* Chicago: Hospital Research and Educational Trust, 1993.

Lanier, J. O., and B. A. Passett. "Innovative Approaches in Governance: A Case Study of the Greater Southeast Healthcare System." *Healthcare Executive* 5, no. 5 (1990): 24–25.

McMahon, J. A. *Creating Community Care Networks: Issues and Opportunities, Report of the 1993 National Forum on Hospitals and Health Affairs, Held in Durham, North Carolina, May 19–21, 1993.* Durham, N.C.: Fuque School of Business, Duke University, 1994.

Newbold, P., and P. Linton. "21st Century Innovators [Interviewed by Joe Flower]." *Healthcare Forum Journal* 35, no. 2 (1992): 70–75.

Orlikoff, James E., and Mary K. Totten. "Trustee Workbook. Assessing and Improving Your Community's Health." *Trustee* 48, no. 5 (1995).

Rice, J. A. *Community Health Assessment: The First Step in Community Health Planning.* Chicago: American Hospital Association, 1993.

Seaman, D. A., B. E. Peters, and C. L. Rugh. "Healthy Communities. Our Focus for the Future." *Michigan Hospitals* 30, no. 5 (1994): 8–13.

Seed, P., and G. Kaye. *Handbook for Assessing and Managing Care in the Community.* London: J. Kingsley, 1994.

Umbdenstock, Richard, Winifred Hageman, and Barry Bader. *Improving and Evaluating Board Performance.* Rockville, Md.: Bader and Associates, 1986.

U.S. Public Health Service. *Starting Points for Creating a Healthy Community.* Washington, D.C.: U.S. Public Health Service and the Department of Health and Human Services, 1994.

VHA, Inc. *Community Partnerships: Taking Charge of Change Through Partnership.* Irving, Tex.: VIIA, Inc., 1993.

VHA, Inc. *Voluntary Community Benefits Standards: A Framework for Meeting Community Health Needs.* Irving, Tex.: VHA, Inc.

VISIONARY LEADERSHIP

Advisory Board Company. *Strategies for Redesigning Care.* Washington, D.C.: The Advisory Board Company, 1991.

"Back on Track: Leading a Hospital Turnaround." *California Hospitals* 7, no. 5 (1993): 10–17.

Barker, Joel Arthur. *Future Edge: Discovering the New Paradigms of Success.* New York: William Morrow, 1992.

Beckhard, Richard, and Wendy Pritchard. *Changing the Essence.* San Francisco: Jossey-Bass, 1992.

Blenden, R. J., and J. N. Edwards, eds. *System in Crisis: The Case for Health Care Reform.* Washington, D.C.: Healthcare Information Center, 1991.

Coile, Russell C., and R. M. Grossman. "Visionary Leadership." *Healthcare Forum Leadership* 31, no. 5 (1988): 42–44.

Davis, P. A. "Unit-Based Shared Governance. Nurturing the Vision." *Journal of Nursing Administration* 22, no. 12 (1992): 46–50.

Ewell, C. M. "A Shared Vision of Hospital Leadership." *Trustee* 43, no. 4 (1990): 12–13.

Fennell, M. L., and J. A. Alexander. "Governing Board and Profound Organizational Change in Hospitals." *Medical Care Review* 46, no. 2 (1989): 157–87.

Fritz, Robert. *Creating.* New York: Fawcett Columbine, 1991.

Heider, John. *The Tao of Leadership.* New York: Bantam, 1985.

Houle, C. O. *Governing Boards: Their Nature and Nurture.* San Francisco: Jossey-Bass, 1989.

Jaeger, B. Jon, ed. *Hospitals in the Year 2000.* Durham, N.C.: Department of Health Administration, Duke University, 1991.

Kotter, John P. *The Leadership Factor.* New York: The Free Press, 1988.

Levin, D. F. "Leadership and Vision." *Emphasis: Nursing* 4, no. 2 (1995): 21–22.

Levinson, Harry, and Stuart Rosenthal. *CEO—Corporate Leadership in Action.* New York: Basic Books, 1984.

Nanus, Burt, and Warren Bennis. *Visionary Leadership: Creating a Compelling Sense of Direction for Your Organization.* San Francisco: Jossey-Bass, 1992.

Peters, Thomas J., and Robert H. Waterman. *In Search of Excellence.* New York: Harper and Row, 1982.

Rindler, M. E. *The Challenge of Hospital Governance: How to Become an Exemplary Board.* Chicago: American Hospital Publishing, 1992.

Ross, A. *Cornerstones of Leadership for Health Services Executives.* Ann Arbor, Mich.: Health Administration Press, 1992.

Schein, E. H. *Organizational Culture and Leadership.* San Francisco: Jossey-Bass, 1990.

Sherman, V. Clayton. *Creating the New American Hospital.* San Francisco: Jossey-Bass, 1993.

Slesinger, L. H. *Self-Assessment for Nonprofit Governing Boards.* Washington, D.C.: National Center for Nonprofit Boards, 1991.

Sobol, M., R. Solum, and B. Wall. *The Visionary Leader: How to Build Leadership, Trust and Participation in Your Company.* Rocklin, Cal.: Prima, 1992.

Tyrrell, R. A. "Visioning: An Important Management Tool." *Nursing Economics* 12, no. 2 (1994): 92, 93–95.

Ulshak, Francis L. *The Common Bond, Maintaining Constancy of Purpose Throughout Your Health Care Organization.* San Francisco: Jossey-Bass, 1984.

Weisbord, Marvin, and others. *Discovering Common Ground.* San Francisco: Berrett-Koehler, 1992.

World Health Organization. *Public Policy for Healthy Cities: Involving the Policy Makers.* Inaugural Conference of the World Health Organization Collaboration Center in Healthy Cities, 1992.

SYSTEMS THINKING

Adizes, Ichak. *Corporate Lifecycles.* Englewood Cliffs, N.J.: Prentice-Hall, 1988.

Alexander, J. A., L. L. Morlock, and B. D. Gifford. "The Effects of Corporate Restructuring on Hospital Policymaking." *Health Services Research* 23, no. 2 (1988): 311–37.

American College of Healthcare Executives and the American Hospital Association. *The Partnership Study: A Study of Rules and Working Relationships of the Hospital Board Chairman, CEO, and Medical Staff President, Survey Findings.* Chicago: ACHE and AHA, 1993.

Andrews, H. A., and others. *Organizational Transformation in Health Care: A Work in Progress.* San Francisco: Jossey-Bass, 1984.

Arnstein, Sherry R. "A Ladder of Citizen Participation." *AIP Journal* (July 1969): 216–24.

Axelrod, N., and others. "The Governance Symposium—Part II. A New Context for Trustees." *Trustee* 47, no. 9 (1994): 10–13.

Blenden, R. J., and M. Brodie, eds. *Transforming the System: Buidling a New Structure for a New Century.* Washington, D.C.: Faulkner and Gray Healthcare Information Center, 1984.

Charns, M. P., and L. J. Smith Tewskbury. *Collaborative Management in Health Care.* San Francisco: Jossey-Bass, 1993.

Coile, Russell C. "Strategic Tools: Part II. Systems Thinking: A New Paradigm for Executive Strategy." *Hospital Strategic Report* 1, no. 10 (1989): 1, 3–4.

Covey, Stephen R. *The 7 Habits of Highly Effective People.* New York: Simon and Shuster, 1989.

Deal, Terrence E., and Allen A. Kennedy. *Corporate Cultures, The Rites and Rituals of Corporate Life.* Reading, Mass.: Addison-Wesley, 1984.

Duhl, B. S. *From the Inside Out and Other Metaphors: Creative and Integrative Approaches to Training in Systems Thinking.* New York: Brunner/Mazel, 1983.

Ferguson, Marilyn. *The Aquarian Conspiracy: Personal and Social Transformation in Our Time.* New York: G. P. Putnam's Sons, 1987.

Gerybadze, A. *Strategic Alliances and Process Redesign: Effective Management and Restructuring of Cooperative Projects and Networks.* New York: Walter De Gruyter, 1994.

Goldstein, D. E. *Alliances: Strategies for Building Integrated Delivery Systems.* Gaithersburg, Md.: Aspen, 1995.

Green, J. "CHC Seeing Fruits of Efforts to Improve Communications." *Modern Healthcare* 22, no. 22 (1992): 38.

Harvard Law School Program on Negotiation. *Annual Report.* Cambridge, Mass.: Program on Negotiation. Annual publication.

Himmelmann, Arthur T. *Collaboration for a Change: Definitions, Models and Roles, with a User Friendly Guide to Collaborative Processes.* Minneapolis: Himmelman Consulting Group, 1995.

"Hospital System Boards Adjust to Changing Roles." *Modern Healthcare* 21, no. 35 (1991): 22–28.

Johnson, E. A., and R. L. Johnson. *New Dynamics for Hospital Boards.* Ann Arbor, Mich.: Health Administration Press, 1994.

Kidder, Rushworth M. *Shared Values For a Troubled World, Conversations with Men and Women of Conscience.* San Francisco: Jossey-Bass, 1994.

Minnen, T. G., and others. "Sustaining Work Redesign Innovations through Shared Governance." *Journal of Nursing Administration* 23, nos. 7–8 (1993): 35–40.

Moss, M. "From Reengineering to Service Integration." *Nursing Management* 25, no. 8 (1994): 80E–80F.

Moss, M., M. Eagen, and M. B. Russell. "Service Integration in the Reform Era." *Nursing Economics* 12, no. 5 (1994): 256–60, 286.

Mott, B. J. *Trusteeship and the Future of Community Hospitals.* Chicago: American Hospital Publishing, 1984.

Motz, D., and J. Lewis. "Shared Governance. Is It a Catalyst of Change?" *Journal of Burn Care and Rehabilitation* 15, no. 4 (1994): 375–85.

Schein, Edgar H. *Organizational Culture and Leadership.* San Francisco: Jossey-Bass, 1990.

Senge, Peter. *The Fifth Discipline: The Art and Practice of the Learning Organization.* New York: Doubleday/Currency, 1990.

Shortell, S. M., and others. "Building Integrated Systems—the Holographic Organization." *Healthcare Forum Journal* 36, no. 2 (1995): 20–26.

Tiffany, B. A. "Structural Alternatives to Increase Managed Care Business and Service Integration." *Behavioral Healthcare Tomorrow* 3, no. 5 (1994): 79–81, 1994.

Totten, Mary K., James E. Orlikoff, and C. M. Ewell. *The Guide to Governance for Hospital Trustees.* Chicago: American Hospital Publishing, 1990.

Watson, T. *A Business and Its Beliefs.* New York: McGraw-Hill, 1963.

HIGH-LEVERAGE ACTIONS

Abendshien, J. *A Guide to the Board's Role in Strategic Business Planning.* Chicago: American Hospital Publishing, 1988.

Alexander, J. A. "Governance for Whom? The Dilemmas of Change and Effectiveness in Hospital Boards." *Frontiers of Health Services Management* 6, no. 3 (1990): 38–41, 46.

Alexander, J. A., and K. A. Schroer. "Governance in Multihospital Systems: an Assessment of Decision-Making Responsibility." *Hospital and Health Services Administration* 30, no. 2 (1985): 9–20.

Andrews, Kenneth R. *The Concept of Corporate Strategy.* Rev. ed. Homewood, Ill.: Richard D. Irwin, 1980.

Assay, L. D., and J. A. Maciariello. *Executive Leadership in Healthcare.* San Francisco: Jossey-Bass, 1991.

Baehr, R. A. *Engineering a Hospital Turnaround.* Chicago: American Hospital Publishing, 1993.

Begun, J. W., and R. C. Lippincott. *Strategic Adaptation in the Health Professions: Meeting the Challenges of Change.* San Francisco: Jossey-Bass, 1993.

Bland, C. J., and M. T. Ruffin. "Characteristics of a Productive Research Environment: Literature Review." *Academic Medicine* 67, no. 6 (1992): 385–97.

Byham, William C. *Zap, The Lightning of Empowerment.* New York: Harmony Books, 1988.

Campbell, C. A. "The Critical Attributes of Leadership." *Topics in Health Information Management* 13, no. 2 (1992): 9–19.

Carver, J. *Boards That Make a Difference: A New Design for Leadership in Nonprofit and Public Organizations.* San Francisco: Jossey-Bass, 1990.

Conrad, D. A., and G. A. Hoare, eds. *Strategic Alignment: Managing Integrated Health Systems.* Arlington, Va.: AUPHA Press, 1994.

Dalzial, M. M., and S. C. Schoonover. *Changing Ways: A Practical Tool for Implementing Change within Organizations.* New York: American Management Association, 1988.

Duncan, W. J., P. M. Ginter, and L. E. Swayne. *Strategic Management for Health Care Organizations.* Boston, Mass.: PWS-Kent, 1992.

Fisher, Roger, and William Ury. *Getting to Yes: Negotiating Agreement without Giving In.* Boston: Houghton Mifflin, 1983.

Gill, S. L., and R. L. Johnson. "Growing Pains: Twelve Lessons from Corporate Restructuring." *Health Progress* 69, no. 4 (1988): 26–32.

Goldman, Ellen F., and Kevin C. Nolan. *Strategic Planning in Health Care: A Guide for Board Members.* Chicago: American Hospital Publishing, 1994.

Goodstein, J., and W. Boeker. "Turbulence at the Top: a New Perspective on Governance Structure Changes and Strategic Change." *Academy of Management Journal* 34, no. 2 (1991): 306–30.

Harris, J. C. *Strategic Health Management: A Guide for Employers, Employees, and Policymakers.* San Francisco: Jossey-Bass, 1994.

Health Care Advisory Board. *Competitive Strategy.* The CEO Series, vol. 2. Washington, D.C.: Health Care Advisory Board, 1990.

King, Bob. *Hoshin Planning: The Developmental Approach.* Methuen, Mass.: GOAL/QPC, 1989.

Leech, J. D. "The Shape of Things to Come: Restructuring Hospitals for the 90's." *Trustee* 45, no. 3 (1992): 4–6.

Mirvis, Phillip H., and Mitchell Lee Marks. *Managing the Merger, Making It Work.* Englewood Cliffs, N.J.: Prentice-Hall, 1992.

"A Model for Strategic Leadership." *Hospital Trustee* 13, no. 4 (1989): 10–12.

Mason, R. O., I. J. Mitroff, and C. M. Pearson. *Framebreak: The Radical Redesign of American Businesses.* San Francisco: Jossey-Bass, 1994.

McWhinney, Will, and others. *Creating Paths of Change.* Venice, Cal.: Enthusion, 1991.

Melum, Mara Minerva, and Casey Collett. *Breakthrough Leadership: Achieving Organizational Alignment through Hoshin Planning.* Chicago: American Hospital Publishing, 1995.

Moses, Richard P. *Evaluation of the Hospital Board and the Chief Executive Officer.* Chicago: American Hospital Publishing, 1986.

Mott, B. J. "Four Critical Areas in Governance." *Hospital Trustee* 9, no. 2 (1985): 7–9.

Norman, F. J. "The Board's Role in Leading Change. Centre for Quality in Governance." *Leadership in Health Services* 2, no. 4 (1993): 36–37.

Pegels, C. C., and K. A. Rodgers. *Strategic Management of Hospitals and Healthcare Facilities.* Rockville, Md.: Aspen, 1988.

Peters, Joseph P., and Simon Tseng. *Managing Strategic Change in Hospitals.* Chicago: American Hospital Publishing, 1983.

Porter, Michael E. *Competitive Strategy.* New York: The Free Press, 1980.

Price, Pritchett. *Making Mergers Work: A Guide to Managing Mergers and Acquisitions.* Homewood, Ill.: Dow Jones-Irwin, 1987.

Primozic, Kenneth, Edward Primozic, and Joe Leben. *Strategic Choices, Supremacy, Survival or Sayonara.* New York: McGraw-Hill, 1991.

Rathwell, T. *Strategic Planning in the Health Sector.* New York: Croom Helm, 1987.

Ries, Al, and Jack Trout. *Marketing Warfare.* New York: McGraw-Hill, 1986.

Ries, Al, and Jack Trout. *Positioning: The Battle for Your Mind.* New York: McGraw-Hill, 1981.

Savage, T. J. "Navigating the System Governance Maze." *Health Progress* 68, no. 1 (1987): 30–37.

Schein, Edgar H. "On Dialogue, Culture, and Organizational Learning." *Organizational Dynamics* 22, no. 2 (1993): 40–51.

Schein, Edgar H. *Process Consultation—Its Role in Organization Development.* Reading, Mass.: Addison-Wesley, 1988.

Seidel, L. F., J. W. Seavey, and R. J. A. Lewis. *Strategic Management for Healthcare Organizations.* Owings Mills, Md.: AUPHA Press, 1989.

Shapiro, Eileen C. *How Corporate Truths Become Competitive Traps.* New York: John Wiley and Sons, 1991.

Shortell, S. M. "New Directions in Hospital Governance." *Hospital & Health Services Administration* 34, no. 1 (1989): 7–23.

Shortell, S. M., E. M. Morrison, and B. Friedman. *Strategic Choices for America's Hospitals: Managing Change in Turbulent Times.* San Francisco: Jossey-Bass, 1990.

Simyar, F., and J. Lloyd-Jones, eds. *Strategic Management in the Health Care Sector.* Englewood Cliffs, N.J.: Prentice-Hall, 1988.

Umbdenstock, Richard, and Winifred Hageman. *Critical Readings for Hospital Trustees.* Chicago: American Hospital Publishing, 1991.

Umbdenstock, Richard, Winifred Hageman, and B. Amundson. "The Five Critical Areas for Effective Governance of Not-for-Profit Hospitals." *Hospital & Health Services Administration* 35, no. 4 (1990): 481–92.

Von Clausewitz, Carl. *On War.* New York: Penguin, 1988.

Von Oech, Roger. *A Whack on the Side of the Head.* New York: Warner, 1983.

Wagner, L. "Change in Governance Urged for D.C. General." *Modern Healthcare* 24, no. 21 (1994): 26.

Wilson, C. K. "Shared Governance: The Challenge of Change in the Early Phases of Implementation." *Nursing Administration Quarterly* 13, no. 4 (1989): 29–33.

Witt, J. A. *Building a Better Hospital Board.* Ann Arbor, Mich.: Health Administration Press, 1987.

BASIC SKILLS

Akao, Yoji, ed. *Quality Function Deployment.* Portland, Ore.: Productivity Press, 1990.

Alexander, J. A., and L. L. Morlock. "CEO-Board Relationships under Hospital Corporate Restructuring." *Hospital & Health Services Administration* 33, no. 4 (1988): 435–48.

Alexander, J. A., and James E. Orlikoff. "Hospital Restructuring Gains Widespread Acceptance." *Trustee* 40, no. 1 (1987): 16–18.

Baehr, Richard A. *Engineering a Hospital Turnaround.* Chicago: American Hospital Publishing, 1993.

Boland, Peter. *Making Managed Healthcare Work, A Practical Guide to Strategies and Solutions.* Gaithersburg, Md.: Aspen, 1993.

Bradford, C. K., and J. F. Tiscornia. *Monitoring the Hospital's Financial Health.* Chicago: American Hospital Publishing, 1987.

Campbell, C. A. "The Critical Attributes of Leadership." *Topics in Health Information Management* 13, no. 2 (1992): 9–19.

Coile, Russell C. *The New Governance: Strategies for an Era of Health Reform.* Ann Arbor, Mich.: Health Administration Press, 1994.

Couch, J. B., and J. M. Juran. *Health Care Quality Management for the 21st Century.* Venice, Fla.: American College of Medical Quality and American College of Physician Executives, 1991.

Crosby, Philip B. *Quality Is Free—The Art of Making Quality Certain.* New York: Penguin, 1980.

Crosby, Philip B. *Running Things: The Art of Making Things Happen.* New York: Penguin Books, 1987.

Doody, M. F. *The Trustee's Guide to Compensation for Healthcare Executives.* Chicago: Probus, 1993.

Ernst & Young Quality Control Improvement Consulting Group. *Total Quality—An Executive's Guide for the 1990s.* Homewood, Ill.: Business One Irwin, 1990.

Hafertepe, E. C. "Systemwide Board Assessment." *Health Progress* 68, no. 1 (1987): 82–86.

Health Care Advisory Board. *Million Dollar Cost Savings Ideas.* The CEO Series, vol. 1. Washington, D.C.: The Health Care Advisory Board, 1989.

Herzlinger, R. E. *Creating New Health Care Ventures: The Role of Management.* Gaithersburg, Md.: Aspen, 1992.

Joint Commission on Accreditation of Healthcare Organizations. *Striving Toward Improvement.* Oakbrook Terrace, Ill.: Joint Commission, 1992.

Kaufman, Kenneth, and Mark L. Hall. *The Capital Management of Health Care Organizations.* Ann Arbor, Mich.: Health Administration Press, 1990.

Kongstvedt, Peter R. *The Managed Health Care Handbook.* Gaithersburg, Md.: Aspen, 1993.

Kovner, A. R. "Improving Hospital Board Effectiveness: An Update." *Frontiers of Health Services Management* 6, no. 3 (1990): 3–27.

Kubeck, L. C. *Techniques for Business Process Redesign: Tying It All Together.* New York: John Wiley and Sons, 1995.

Moore, Terence F., and Earl A. Simendinger. *Hospital Turnarounds: Lessons in Leadership.* Ann Arbor, Mich.: Health Administration Press, 1993.

Moses, R. P. *Evaluation of the Hospital Board and the Chief Executive Officer.* Chicago: American Hospital Publishing, 1986.

Mott, B. J. "Four Critical Areas in Governance." *Hospital Trustee* 9, no. 2 (1985): 7–9.

National Forum on Hospital and Health Affairs. *Improving Hospital Decisionmaking: Report of the 1988 National Forum on Hospital and Health Affairs, Held in Durham, North Carolina, May 12–14, 1988.* Washington, D.C.: Department of Health Administration, 1989.

Orlikoff, James E. *Quality from the Top: Working with Hospital Governing Boards to Assure Quality Care.* Chicago: Pluribus Press, 1990.

Orlikoff, James E., and Mary K. Totten. *The Board's Role in Quality Care.* Chicago: American Hospital Publishing, 1991.

Savage, T. J. "Navigating the System Governance Maze." *Health Progress* 68, no. 1 (1979): 30–37.

Shortell, S. M., and U. E. Reinhardt. *Improving Health Policy and Management: Nine Critical Research Issues for the 1990s.* Ann Arbor, Mich.: AHSR/Health Administration Press, 1992.

Stevens, G. H. *The Strategic Health Care Manager: Mastering Essential Leadership Skills.* San Francisco: Jossey-Bass, 1991.

Taylor, S. B., and R. J. Taylor. *The AUPHA Manual of Health Services Management.* Gaithersburg, Md.: Aspen, 1994.

Tomasko, Robert M. *Downsizing: Reshaping the Corporation for the Future.* New York: AMACOM, 1987.

Walton, Mary. *Deming Management at Work.* New York: G. P. Putnam's Sons, 1990.

Walton, Mary. *The Deming Management Method.* New York: G. P. Putnam's Sons, 1986.

Yasuda, Yuzo. *Forty Years, 20 Million Ideas: The Toyota Suggestion System.* Portland, Ore.: Productivity Press, 1990.

Zander, A. *Making Boards Effective: The Dynamics of Nonprofit Governing Boards.* San Francisco: Jossey-Bass, 1993.

Zemke, Ron. *The Service Edge: 101 Companies That Profit from Customer Care.* New York: Penguin, 1990.

Index